Respiratory pocket

Author: Dževad Bajraktarević , R.R.T.-N.P.S., Michael Jakob, M.D.
Editor: Carla Maute, M.D., Gabriele Keller
Production: Sylvia Engel
Publisher: Börm Bruckmeier Publishing LLC, www.media4u.com

© 2004–2006, by **Börm Bruckmeier Publishing LLC**
68 17th Street, Hermosa Beach, CA 90254
www.media4u.com
Second Edition

IMPORTANT NOTICE – PLEASE READ!
This book is based on information from sources believed to be reliable, and every effort ha been made to make the book as complete and accurate as possible and to describe generall accepted practices based on information available as of the printing date, but its accuracy and completeness cannot be guaranteed. Despite the best efforts of author and publisher, the book may contain errors, and the reader should use the book only as a general guide and not as the ultimate source of information about the subject matter.
This book is not intended to reprint all of the information available to the author or publisher on the subject, but rather to simplify, complement and supplement other availabl sources. The reader is encouraged to read all available material and to consult the package insert and other references to learn as much as possible about the subject.
This book is sold without warranties of any kind, expressed or implied, and the publisher an author disclaim any liability, loss or damage caused by the content of this book.
IF YOU DO NOT WISH TO BE BOUND BY THE FOREGOING CAUTIONS AND CONDITIONS , YO MAY RETURN THIS BOOK TO THE PUBLISHER FOR A FULL REFUND.

Printed in China
ISBN 1-59103-228-8

Preface

Respiratory pocket is a clinical reference guide offering quick access to definitive diagnosis and treatment information for all types of respiratory diseases.

It is intended for physicians, pulmonologists, respiratory care physicians, medical students, and all healthcare professionals.

The format of the text is user-friendly. We use an outline-style structure with diagrams and numerous tables and illustrations to allow the reader easy access to, and assimilation of, the information provided. Inevitably, a book of this size will not be comprehensive, but even massive encyclopedic textbooks cannot cover every aspect of pulmonary medicine and respiratory care.

Nevertheless, we have attempted to cover as much material as possible, and we sincerely hope that you will enjoy this book and that it will be of great help to you.

We gladly welcome any criticism, suggestions, and/or ideas that you think could improve this book. Please write to us at service@media4u.com.

Dževad Bajraktarević   July 2004
Michael Jakob

DEDICATION

To my beautiful wife Michele and son Jenan.

Dževad Bajraktarević

6 Content

8 Content

ANATOMY AND PHYSIOLOGY OF THE RESPIRATORY SYSTEM

1.   Anatomy

1.1   Upper Airways

1.1.1   Nose

Functions: warms, humidifies and filters out particles > 5-10 μm;
conducts air to lower respiratory tract; olfaction

1.1.2   Pharynx

Subdivided into:

Nasopharynx
Extends from posterior nares to uvula. Contains Eustachian tubes and adenoids
(pharyngeal tonsils), which if inflamed may block Eustachian tubes leading to
otitis media (ear infection)

Oropharynx
Extends from uvula to epiglottis. Contains lingual tonsils (base of tongue; anterior
oropharyngeal wall) and palatine tonsils (lateral oropharynx), which if inflamed
may lead to airway obstruction

Laryngopharynx
Extends from epiglottis to vocal cords/esophagus. Contains epiglottis and uvula,
which are intubation points

1.1.3   Larynx

Located at the level of the 4th - 6th cervical vertebrae (epiglottis to trachea).
Composed of 9 cartilages, 3 single and 3 paired:

Single cartilages

Epiglottis:
Diverts food into esophagus by covering glottis during swallowing

Glottis:

Opening into larynx, formed by vocal cords = narrowest point in adult's upper airway.
It is innervated by vagus nerve via laryngeal nerve and injury to it possibly
⇒ speech loss ± dysphagia

Thyroid:

Largest cartilage; also known as Adam's apple

Cricoid:

The only cartilage that fully encircles airway
It is the narrowest point in infant's upper airway

Paired cartilages

Arytenoids:

Vocal cords attach to them; along with cricoid cartilage, make up the entire posterior
surface of the larynx

Corniculates:

Provide structural support for arytenoids

Cuneiforms:

Attached to arytenoids; shaped like small elongated clubs

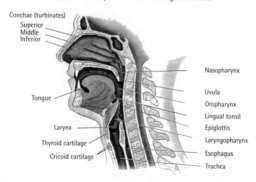

Fig. 1 Cross-sectional view showing major structures of upper airways

1.2 Lower Airways

There are about 23 - 27 airway generations.

1.2.1 Generations

Trachea (0)

Extends from the cricoid cartilage to the carina. Contains ~ 15 - 20 C-shaped cartilages. Posteriorly, it is separated from the esophagus by the trachealis muscle. The trachea is ~ 12 cm long and 1.5 - 2.5 cm wide in adults and ~ 7 cm long in infants. The trachea bifurcates into right and left main-stem bronchi at the carina.

Main-stem bronchi (1)

Right main-stem bronchus:

Forms 20 - 30° angle. It is ~ 1.5 cm wide and 2.5 cm long and a less acute angle than the left main-stem bronchi ⇒ ↑ risk of aspiration in the right lung

Left main-stem bronchus:

Forms 45 - 55° angle. It is ~ 1 cm wide and 5 cm long

Lobar bronchi (2)

Right main-stem bronchus trifurcates into upper, middle and lower bronchi (lobes) and left main-stem bronchus divides into upper and lower bronchi

Segmental bronchi (3)

18 segmental bronchi correspond to 18 lung segments: 10 in the right and 8 in left lung

> **NOTE:** Some authorities consider that the left lung also has 10 segments, with segments 1 and 2 and segments 7 and 8 being fused.

Small bronchi (4 - 9)

Diameter decreases from ~ 4 mm to 1 mm. Very little cartilage is present by the 9th generation.

1.2.2 Start of non-cartilagenous 'small' airways

Bronchioles (10 - 15)

These airways are < 1 mm in diameter and conduct gas to the area of gas exchange. Since they lack supporting cartilage, they are susceptible to bronchospasm and ↑ airway resistance (R_{aw}).

Terminal bronchioles (16 - 19)

Lack goblet cells, glands and cilia. Diameter is ~ 0.5 mm; terminal bronchioles mark the **end of conducting airways** (dead space ≈ $\frac{1}{3}$ of V_T)

1.2.3 Start of gas exchange area

Respiratory bronchioles (20 - 23)

Mark the beginning of the respiratory zone = **start of alveoli** (lung parenchyma). Diameter is ~ 0.5 mm

Alveolar ducts (24 - 26)

Arise from respiratory bronchioles. Each duct ends in clusters of alveoli

Alveolar sacs (27)

Grapelike clusters of 10 - 20 alveoli with common walls. This is the final generation of airways

Alveoli

There are ~ 300 million alveoli in the lungs and the number is directly proportional to body height. Each alveolus is surrounded by hundreds of capillaries, covering ~ 90% of the alveolar wall = huge gas exchange area of ~ 75 m^2 (size of tennis court). Alveoli are composed of:

Type I alveolar cells:

Squamous, thin and flat covering ~ 95% of alveolar surface

Type II alveolar cells:

Cuboidal, granular cells that produce surfactant, which prevents alveolar collapse. They cover only ~ 5% of alveolar surface but are more numerous than type I cells

Macrophages:

Phagocytize foreign material that reaches alveoli. They do not originate in the lungs

Alveolar–capillary (A-C) membrane

Gas exchange area; it is ~ 1 - 2 μm thick and is made up of surfactant, alveolar epithelium, interstitial space and capillary endothelium. For O_2 to get from alveolus to hemoglobin (Hb), it must cross A-C membrane + plasma, red blood cell (RBC) membrane and RBC cytoplasm.

Collateral ventilatory channels

Pores of Kohn:

Small holes in the interalveolar septa, which allow collateral air movement between adjacent alveoli. They are ~ 5 - 15 μm in size and their number and size increases progressively with age and disease (e.g. chronic obstructive pulmonary disease; COPD)

Canals of Lambert:

Small channels connecting respiratory bronchioles and adjacent alveoli. They are ~ 30 μm in size

> *NOTE: The pores of Kohn and canals of Lambert may be important in shunting air around an obstruction (COPD) to reach perfused alveoli.*

1.3   Lungs

The lungs weigh ~ 800 g in adults. Composed of ~ 10% tissue and 90% gas + blood. **Apex** is the top of the lung, which rises to about the level of the clavicles or ~ 2 cm higher. **Base** is the bottom of the lung, which lies on the diaphragm, 6th rib anteriorly and 10th rib posteriorly.

1.3.1   Right lung

Composed of 3 lobes (upper, middle, lower) and 10 segments. It is heavier and shorter than the left lung due to the liver pushing up on right hemidiaphragm.

1.3.2   Left lung

Composed of 2 lobes (upper, lower) and 8 segments. It is narrower than the right lung due to the heart protruding to the left.

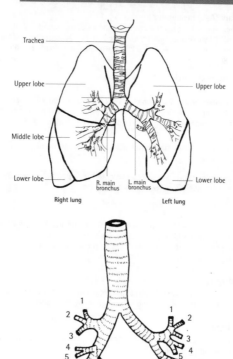

Fig. 2 Anterior view of the lungs and the bronchial tree

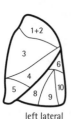
left lateral

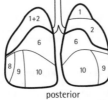
anterior

right lateral

left medial

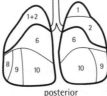
posterior

right medial

Left lung:
Upper lobe
1 + 2 Apical
3 Anterior
4 Sup. segment of lingula
5 Inf. segment of lingula
Lower lobe
6 Superior
7 + 8 Ant.-med. basal
9 Lat. basal
10 Post. basal

Right lung:
Upper lobe
1 Apical
2 Posterior
3 Anterior
Middle lobe
4 Lateral
5 Medial
Lower lobe
6 Superior
7 Med. basal   9 Lat. basal
8 Ant. basal   10 Post. basal

Fig. 3 Segments of the lungs

1.4   Pleura

1.4.1   Parietal pleura
Lines the inner layer of thorax. Has nerve endings for pain sensation

1.4.2   Visceral pleura
Lines the lungs

1.4.3   Intrapleural space
Potential space between parietal and visceral pleurae, which is occupied by thin layer of fluid (< 15 ml) allowing pleurae to slide over each other. If air or fluid enters this space, pleurae will separate, which ⇒ PTX or pleural effusion.

1.5   Thorax
Encloses/protects organs within it (heart, vessels, lungs, stomach, liver, spleen) and provides attachments for respiratory muscles. Thoracic cage is composed of the sternum anteriorly and ribs and thoracic vertebrae posteriorly.

1.5.1   Sternum
Forms the anterior border of the chest. It is ~ 18 cm long and is composed of 3 sections: manubrium (upper part), body (middle part) and xiphoid process (lower cartilaginous part). Angle of Louis is a junction between body and manubrium; it serves as an anatomical landmark for the carina.

1.5.2   Ribs
12 ribs correspond to 12 thoracic vertebrae. Note that procedures such as thoracentesis must be performed above the rib, because intercostal nerves, veins and arteries lie below each rib. The space between each rib (intercostal space) contains intercostal muscles.

True ribs
1st 7 ribs; connect directly to sternum via costal cartilages

False ribs
Ribs 8 - 10; their cartilage attaches to cartilage of 1st 7 ribs

Floating ribs
Ribs 11 - 12; not connected to sternum and float free

1.6 Respiratory Muscles

1.6.1 Inspiratory muscles

Diaphragm
This is the main respiratory muscle and is responsible for > 75% of ventilation during normal quiet breathing. It is innervated by the phrenic nerve (C3, 4, 5), which splits to innervate both hemidiaphragms. If the phrenic nerve is injured, this may ⇒ diaphragmatic paralysis. Right hemidiaphragm is slightly higher than left due to liver being under it. Structures that pass through the diaphragm: aorta, inferior vena cava (IVC), esophagus and major nerves.

Accessory muscles of inspiration
These muscles assist the diaphragm during ↑ ventilatory demand. Include external intercostals, scalenes, sternocleidomastoid, trapezius and pectoralis minor and major.

1.6.2 Expiratory muscles

Accessory muscles of expiration
Expiration is normally passive due to elastic recoil of lungs and chest wall. Active expiration may occur in exercise and COPD patients. Includes abdominal muscles and intercostals.

1.7 Lung Defenses

1.7.1 Nasal hairs/turbinates

Filter out particles > 5 - 10 μm in diameter; particles impact on mucous membrane due to turbulent airflow

1.7.2 Reflexes

Cough
Due to stimulation of receptors in larynx and trachea (esp. carina); inhibited by anesthesia

Sneeze
Due to stimulation of nasopharynx; in both reflexes, explosive expiration is likely to remove mucus and irritant

1.7.3 Mucus & mucociliary escalator

Mucus

Traps, filters out inspired particles

Mucociliary escalator

Cilia beat ~ 20 x/s and push mucus + trapped particles up to oropharynx to be swallowed or coughed out. Cilia are inhibited by anesthesia, smoking, endotracheal tube, high FIO_2 and ↑ volume and thickness of mucus. Goblet cells and submucosal glands ↑ in number during irritation (e.g. COPD) ⇒ ↑ mucus production. Submucosal glands are innervated by parasympathetic nervous system and parasympathetic drugs (e.g. atropine) ↓ secretion production.

1.7.4 Alveolar macrophages

Engulf/destroy bacteria or particles that evade mucociliary escalator/mucus and reach lung parenchyma

1.8 Lung Innervation

1.8.1 Sympathetic nervous system (SNS)

- Stimulation of SNS causes bronchodilation when neurotransmitters such as epinephrine are secreted by adrenal gland and released onto airway muscle; this activates β_2 adrenergic receptors ⇒ bronchodilation
- Produces thin secretions: β_2 agonists such as albuterol stimulate SNS to produce bronchodilation

1.8.2 Parasympathetic nervous system (PNS)

- Stimulation (via vagus nerve) causes release of acetylcholine (Ach) on to airway smooth muscle, causing bronchoconstriction, vasodilation and ↑ mucus production
- Anticholinergics such as ipratropium bromide (Atrovent) are used to block this effect

1.9 Lung Circulation

1.9.1 Bronchial circulation

Small branch of systemic circulation **supplying** tracheobronchial tree (down to terminal bronchioles) with oxygenated blood and nutrients
- **Origin:** aorta + intercostal arteries
- **Drainage:** via pulmonary veins into left heart, which contributes to normal anatomical shunt of 1 - 2% of cardiac output (CO)

1.9.2 Pulmonary circulation

- Carries mixed venous blood (deoxygenated) from tissues to lungs to pick up oxygen and eliminate carbon dioxide
- Low resistance, low pressure & high compliance system (pulmonary vascular resistance [PVR] is ~ $\frac{1}{10}$ of systemic vascular resistance [SVR])
- Right ventricle (RV) pumps deoxygenated blood via pulmonary artery (PA) to A-C membrane, where gas exchange occurs. Oxygenated blood is carried by pulmonary veins to left ventricle (LV) to be pumped throughout body
- Normally, CO is ~ 5 L/min at rest, but can ↑ to > 20 L/min in exercise. Blood volume in pulmonary capillaries is normally ~ 75 - 150 ml, but can ↑ to > 250 ml in exercise

1.9.3 Distribution of pulmonary blood flow: Lung zones

Uneven within lung due to: (1) **gravity:** blood flow is greatest in gravity-dependent areas; (2) **low pressure system:** low PVR as compared to SVR. Lung zones have been recommended to more easily understand the effects on regional blood flow in the lungs. These zones are divided into 3 zones based on arterial, venous and alveolar pressures.

Zone 1

This zone (near apex) is normally nonexistent, but may occur in certain conditions. It may be caused by ↓ arterial pressure (P_{art}), such as from shock or hemorrhage or ↑ alveolar pressure (P_{alv}) due to excessive positive pressure ventilation (↑ PPV):

$$P_{alv} > P_{art} > P_{ven}$$

Zone 2

Middle lung region with intermittent blood flow (during systole). P_{art} is greater than P_{alv}, which means that blood flow will occur past alveoli.

$$P_{art} > P_{alv} > P_{ven}$$

Zone 3

Zone 3 is the lung base, where there is constant blood flow and where most of the gas exchange occurs. Perfusion is greater in this region because of gravitational forces.

$$P_{art} > P_{ven} > P_{alv}$$

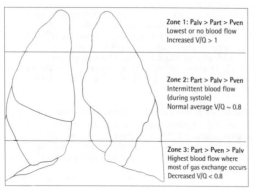

Zone 1: $P_{alv} > P_{art} > P_{ven}$
Lowest or no blood flow
Increased V/Q > 1

Zone 2: $P_{art} > P_{alv} > P_{ven}$
Intermittent blood flow
(during systole)
Normal average V/Q ~ 0.8

Zone 3: $P_{art} > P_{ven} > P_{alv}$
Highest blood flow where
most of gas exchange occurs
Decreased V/Q < 0.8

Fig. 4 Distribution of pulmonary blood flow

2. Physiology

2.1 Ventilation

Minute ventilation (V_E)
$V_E = V_T \times RR$; or $V_E = V_A + V_D$

Alveolar ventilation (V_A)
$V_A = (V_T - V_D) \times RR$; ~ $\frac{2}{3}$ of V_E enters alveoli

Dead space ventilation (V_D)
~ $\frac{1}{3}$ of V_T remains in conductive airways and does not reach alveoli; usually expressed as V_D/V_T ratio (normal: 0.25 - 0.35); contributes to V_E, not V_A; 3 types:

- **$V_D$phys**: = $V_D$anat + $V_D$alv; total volume not involved in gas exchange; normally = $V_D$anat since $V_D$alv is a rare cause of V_D
- **$V_D$anat**: volume in conducting airways; ~ 25 - 35% of V_T; estimated 1 ml/lb of ideal body weight (IBW) (150 lb ≈ 150 ml $V_D$anat)
- **$V_D$alv**: ventilated, nonperfused alveoli; rare cause of V_D; e.g. pulmonary embolism, excessive PPV, ↓ CO

2.2 Ventilation – Perfusion (V/Q) Relationship

2.2.1 Normal V/Q ratio

Ratio of alveolar ventilation (V_A) to pulmonary blood flow or perfusion (Q) normally = 0.8 for entire lung (not region); with an average V_A of 4 L/min and average pulmonary blood flow of 5 L/min (CO)
V/Q = 0.8 (4/5 = 0.8)

2.2.2 Regional V/Q differences in upright lung

Apex
(Zone 1): ↑ V/Q (> 1): = ↑ P_AO_2, ↓ P_ACO_2
Middle
(Zone 2): normal V/Q (0.8): = average P_AO_2, P_ACO_2
Base
(Zone 3): ↓ V/Q: ↓ P_AO_2, ↑ P_ACO_2

2.3   Diffusion of Gases

2.3.1 O_2 cascade

PO_2 pathway from atmosphere to tissues
(at sea level: barometric pressure [Pb] 760 mmHg)

Air $PO_2 \sim 160$ mmHg: $PIO_2 = 760 \times 0.21 = 159$ mmHg [dry inspired air]

⇓

Conductive airways/Trachea $PO_2 \sim 150$ mmHg:
$PIO_2 = (760 - 47) \times 0.21 = 150$ mmHg [humidification: $PH_2O = 47$ mmHg]

⇓

Alveoli $P_AO_2 \sim 105$ mmHg: $P_AO_2 = (713 \times 0.21) - 45 = 105$ mmHg;
PO_2 decreases because CO_2 diffuses into alveoli to be exhaled

⇓

Pulmonary capillary $PcO_2 \sim 100$ mmHg

⇓

Artery $PaO_2 \sim 95$ mmHg: O_2 moves across A-C membrane, creating alveolar to
arterial oxygen tension (A-a) gradient; PO_2 decreases due to CO_2 diffusing into
alveoli; A-a gradient increases with shunt

⇓

Veins $PvO_2 \sim 40$ mmHg = mixed venous O_2; residual after
O_2 transfer to cells

⇓

Mitochondria $PO_2 \sim 3 - 20$ mmHg; = metabolism

NOTE: ↑ *Altitude = smaller values = smaller values as a result of* ↓ *Pb; size of any step may* ↑ *due to pathology.*

2.3.2 Laws of diffusion of gases

Fick's law

Describes factors that determine rate of gas diffusion through the A–C membrane. States that diffusion of gas across A–C membrane is directly proportional to area of membrane, pressure of gas across membrane and diffusion coefficient and inversely proportional to tissue thickness.

$$V_{gas} = [A \times D (P1 - P2)] / T$$

Where,

V_{gas} = gas volume diffusing through A–C membrane (ml/min)
A = surface area of the membrane; in healthy average size adult, this is ~ 70 m^2
D = diffusion coefficient of the gas in the A–C membrane
T = thickness of the tissue barrier; A–C membrane diffusion barrier is $\sim 0.2 - 0.5$ mm; T can ↑ in interstitial edema or fibrosis
P1 – P2 = pressure difference of gas across the membrane

Henry's law

Amount of gas dissolved in a liquid is directly proportional to partial pressure of gas; solubility coefficient (SC) for O_2 = 0.024 ml/mmHg/ml H_2O and for CO_2 = 0.592 ml/mmHg/ml H_2O, so if SC were to be the only factor, then CO_2 $\sim$ 24 x more soluble than O_2 in H_2O [0.592/0.024 = 24]

Graham's law

Gas diffusion is directly proportional to the square root of its molecular weight (MW) and directly proportional to SC; MW for O_2 = 32 and for CO_2 = 44; O_2 is lighter than CO_2 and moves 1.17 x faster than CO_2 (if SC were not to be a factor); ($\sqrt{44} \div \sqrt{32}$ = 6.6 ÷ 5.6 = 1.17); combined effects of both SC and MW (combined Graham and Henry law) = CO_2 diffuses $\sim$ 20 x faster than O_2

$$\frac{5.6 \times 0.592}{6.6 \times 0.024} = \frac{20}{1}$$

2.3.3 Speed of diffusion of gas across A–C membrane

- At resting CO, RBC spends ~ 0.75 s in the pulmonary capillaries and both O_2 and CO_2 equilibrate across membrane in ~ 0.25 s
- At heavy exercise, equilibration occurs in ~ 0.25 s

2.3.4   Pressure gradients: Responsible for gas movement

P_ACO_2, $PaCO_2 = 40$ mmHg and $PvCO_2 = 46$ mmHg $\Rightarrow$ pressure gradient of 6 mmHg

$P_AO_2 = 100$ and $PaO_2 = 95$ mmHg $\Rightarrow$ pressure gradient of 5 mmHg

At high altitude, O_2 is still 21% but Pb is less, which results in lower PO_2:

(1) Sea level: 760 mmHg x 0.21 = 160 mmHg
(2) Denver: 640 mmHg x 0.21 = 134 mmHg
(3) Andes: 380 mmHg x 0.21 = 80 mmHg
(4) Mt Everest: 252 mmHg x 0.21 = 53 mmHg

2.3.5   Diffusion lung capacity (DL)

Description

Rate of gas transfer across A-C membrane. Carbon monoxide (D_LCO) is used to measure this because it combines ~ 210 x faster than O_2 to Hb and does not exert partial pressure in blood plasma. DL measures effectiveness of A-C membrane.

Interpretation

Normal D_LCO	25 ml/min/mmHg ($\uparrow$ ~ 3 x in exercise)
Decreased	emphysema, alveolar filling (pneumonia, edema), interstitial lung disease (ILD), lung resection, $\downarrow$ pulmonary blood flow, $\downarrow$ hematocrit (Hct), $\downarrow V_A$, pulmonary hypertension (PH)
Increased	$\uparrow$ pulmonary blood flow (exercise, pulmonary hemorrhage), $\uparrow$ Hb (polycythemia), supine position due to $\uparrow$ V/Q matching, $\uparrow$ body size (= $\uparrow$ lung size/volume)

2.4   Mechanics of Respiration

2.4.1   Pressures

Barometric pressure (P_b)
Normally 0 (760 mmHg at sea level) unless PPV applied

Airway opening pressure (P_{ao})
Usually atmospheric unless +ve or -ve pressure is applied to the airway

Pleural pressure (P_{pl})
Usually -ve (e.g. subatmospheric) during quiet breathing

2.4.2 Gradients

Chest wall pressure (P_cw)
Pressure gradient across chest wall
$[P_{cw} = P_{pl} - P_b]$

Transpulmonary pressure (PL)
Pressure across lungs; PL is the pressure diference that maintains alveolar inflation
$[PL = P_{alv} - P_{pl}]$

Transrespiratory pressure (P_rs)
Gradient driving airflow into lungs
$[P_{rs} = P_{alv} - P_b]$

Pressure gradient (cmH$_2$O)	Inspiration	Expiration
$P_{cw} = P_{pl} - P_b$	$-5 \Rightarrow -8$	$-8 \Rightarrow -5$
$PL = P_{alv} - P_{pl}$	$+5 \Rightarrow +8$	$+8 \Rightarrow +5$
$P_{rs} = P_{alv} - P_b$	$0 \Rightarrow -3 \Rightarrow 0$	$0 \Rightarrow +3 \Rightarrow 0$

2.4.3 Lung compliance (CL)

Description

Measure of lung stretchability (and chest wall). $[C = DV/DP]$ Inverse of elastance (E) = ability to return to original shape after being stretched

↑ E, ↓ CL = stiffer lungs: fibrosis, edema, etc.
↑ CL, ↓ E = ↓ stiffness: emphysema

Static compliance (C_st): measured under static (no flow) conditions	
Normal	100 ml/cmH$_2$O
Intubated normal	> 60 ml/cmH$_2$O
Equation	$[C_{st} = V_T/(P_{plat} - PEEP)]$
Dynamic compliance (C_dyn): measured at active breathing (airflow)	
Normal	> 40 ml/cmH$_2$O in mechanically ventilated patients
Equation	$[C_{dyn} = V_T/(PIP - PEEP)]$

PIP = positive inspiratory pressure
PEEP = positive end-expiratory pressure

2.4.4   Airway resistance (R_{aw})

Definition
Airflow resistance caused by friction between airflow and airway wall

Equation
R_{aw} = DP/flow in L/s

Normal
0.5 - 2.5 cmH$_2$O/L/s

Distribution
- upper airways ~ 50%
- large airways ~ 30%
- small airways (< 2 mm diam) ~ 20%

↑R_{aw}
↑ airway length, ↑ gas viscosity, ↓ airway diameter. ↓ radius by ½ = ↑ R_{aw} by 16-fold (Poiseuille's law), which can be secondary to secretions, bronchospasm, or airway inflammation

2.5   Control of Respiration

2.5.1   Chemical control

Central chemoreceptors
In medulla stimulated by
↑ PaCO$_2$ = ↑ V$_E$: ↑ V$_T$ ± RR

Peripheral chemoreceptors
(Aortic bodies in arch of aorta; carotid bodies in bifurcation of carotid arteries) stimulated by ↑ PaCO$_2$ and ↓ PaO$_2$ < 60 mmHg = ↑ V$_E$: ↑ RR

NOTE: Medullary chemoreceptors may adapt to chronic CO$_2$ retainers, so remaining drive to breathe is via stimulation of peripheral chemoreceptors by ↓ PaO$_2$.

2.5.2   Central (neural) control (respiratory center)

Dorsal respiratory group (DRG)
Located in dorsal medulla of mainly inspiratory neurons

Ventral respiratory group (VRG)
Located in ventrolateral medulla of both inspiratory and expiratory neurons

Pneumotaxic center
Located in superior pons; neurons inhibit inspiratory neurons?

2.5.3 Reflex control (mechanoreceptors)

Hering-Breuer reflex
(Slowly adapting stretch receptors; SAR)
Location:
Walls of bronchi and bronchioles
Stimulus:
Overinflated lungs (V_T > 1 L as in exercise); overstretched receptors send inhibitory
signals via vagus nerve to DRG to stop further inspiration

Irritant receptors
(Rapidly adapting receptors; RAR)
Location:
Between epithelial cells lining airways
Stimulus:
Inhaled noxious substances, cold air $\Rightarrow$ cough, hyperpnea, bronchospasm,
↑ secretions

Juxtacapillary (J) receptors
Location:
Alveolar walls (interstitium next to capillaries)
Stimulus:
↑ interstitial volume (edema, congestion) $\Rightarrow$ rapid, shallow breathing

BIBLIOGRAPHY

DesJardins T: Cardiopulmonary Anatomy and Physiology: Essentials for
Respiratory Care, 4th ed. Delmar Publishers, 2002.

Lumb AB: Nunn's Applied Respiratory Physiology, 6th ed. Elsevier, 2005.

Levitzky MG: Pulmonary Physiology, 6th ed. New York, McGraw-Hill
Health Publications, 2003.

West JB: Respiratory Physiology: The Essentials, 6th ed. Williams and
Wilkins, 2000.

ASSESSMENT AND MONITORING

3.   History and Physical Examination

3.1   Vital Signs

Temperature (T)	
Normal value	**37°C (98.6°F)**; Range: 36.5 - 37.5°C; daily variation = 0.5°C
Hyperthermia	> 38°C: Infection, fever, exercise; ↓ T = ↑ metabolism = ↑ VO_2, VCO_2 (1°C ↑ = ↑ VO_2 by ~ 10%)
Hypothermia	< 37°C: cold, trauma to hypothalamus
Heart rate (HR)	
Normal value	Adult: **60 - 100 beats/min**; Child: 80 - 120 beats/min; Newborn: 120 -160 beats/min
Tachycardia	> 100 beats/min; causes: hypoxemia, anxiety, pain, fever, hypotension, exercise, side effects of certain drugs
Bradycardia	< normal; causes: hypothermia, heart disease, physically fit
Blood pressure (BP)	
Normal value	Adult: **120/80 mmHg**; Child: 100/65 mmHg, Newborn: 55/38 mmHg
Hypertension (adults)	> 140/90 mmHg; causes: vasoconstriction, stress, family history, ↑ Na, ↑ risk with obesity
Hypotension (adults)	< 90/60 mmHg; causes: shock, hypovolemia, heart disease
Respiratory rate (RR)	
Normal value	Adult: **12 - 20/min**; Child: 20 - 30/min; Newborn: 30 - 60/min

| Tachypnea | > normal; causes: hypoxemia, anxiety, fever, pain, ↓ BP, restrictive lung disease |
| Bradypnea | < normal; causes: hypothermia, head injury, drug overdose (OD) |

3.2 Respiratory Breathing Patterns

Pattern	Characteristics/Some Causes
Eupnea	Normal physiologic breathing; in adults = 12 - 20 breaths/min
Tachypnea	RR > normal: hypotension, anxiety, fever, hypoxemia, restrictive lung disease
Bradypnea	RR < normal: drug OD, sleep, CNS lesions, ↑ ICP
Hyperpnea	Deep breathing (↑ V_T) with normal RR: hypoxia, fever, anxiety
Hypopnea	Shallow breathing (↓ V_T) with normal RR: hypothermia, sleep, sedation
Hyperventilation	↑ V_E and V_A by ↑ RR ± hyperpnea: hypoxemia, hypotension, lung disease, head injury
Hypoventilation	↓ V_A caused by ↓ RR ± hypopnea: sedation, neuromuscular (NM) disease, hypothyroidism
Apnea	Cessation of breathing: sleep apnea, brain injury, CP arrest
Cheyne - Stokes	Breaths ↑ & ↓ in depth & rate with apnea periods of ~ 20 s: CHF
Biot's	Irregular breathing with periods of apnea: meningitis, ↑ ICP, brainstem dysfunction
Kussmaul's	Hyperpnea + tachypnea: metabolic acidosis (DKA), renal failure
Apneustic	Sustained inspiratory pause (↑ Ti): lesions in respiratory center

3.3   Chest Shape

Normal chest has larger lateral than A-P diameter;
In adults, the ratio of A-P to lateral diameter ~ 1:2

Abnormal chest shapes

Barrel chest:
A-P diameter ~ 1:1; associated with COPD (emphysema)

Pectus carinatum: (Pigeon chest)
Sternum displaced anteriorly

Pectus excavatum: (Funnel chest)
Depression of the lower sternum

Kyphosis:
'Hunchback' appearance due to spine curvature

Scoliosis:
Lateral spine curvature

Kyphoscoliosis:
Kyphosis + scoliosis = distortion of lungs

3.4   Use of Accessory Muscles

During advanced stages of COPD, **accessory muscles of inspiration** are often used to assist diaphragm; include scalenes, sternocleidomastoid, pectoralis major and trapezius; **accessory muscles of expiration** are used by severe COPD patients to help lungs deflate; include abdominal muscles and intercostals.

3.5   Cyanosis

- Bluish color of tissue (skin, lips, earlobes, nail beds) caused by > 5 g/dl of deoxyhemoglobin (unsaturated) in the blood
- UNRELIABLE clinical sign if used itself
  (especially with ANEMIC, POLYCYTHEMIC patients)
- NOT an accurate measure of patient's oxygenation; does not always accompany hypoxemia; may also be present in the absence of hypoxemia:
  (1) **Anemic patient** may be hypoxic but not cyanotic; for example: if anemic patient has 6 g of Hb, 50% saturation will give us only 3 g deoxyhemoglobin
  (2) **Polycythemic patients** may be cyanotic but not hypoxemic because they have high quantity of saturated Hb (normal CaO_2)

3.6 Finger Clubbing

Description

Asymptomatic thickening of the fingers; Skin - nail angle is normally < 160°, while in clubbing of fingers it is > 180°

Etiology

Unknown; may be partly due to chronic hypoxemia: COPD, lung cancer, cyanotic congenital heart disease and sarcoidosis, where there is chronic decrease in oxygen supply to tissue

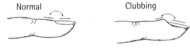

Normal   Clubbing

Fig. 5 'Clubbing'

3.7 Peripheral Edema

Most commonly seen in the ankles and feet due to fluid leaking from capillaries into tissues; most commonly seen in congestive heart failure (CHF) patients; Pitting edema is graded as +1 for 1 mm indention when pressed with finger, +2 for 2 mm etc.

3.8 Jugular Venous Distention (JVD)

↑ venous distention is noted when veins distend above the clavicle when patient's head of bed (HOB) elevation is 30 - 45°; seen in patients with right heart failure (RHF) (cor pulmonale), fluid overload, COPD and high ventilatory pressures during mechanical ventilation (MV)

3.9 Capillary Refill

Pink color of the nail bed should return in < 3 s after it has been pinched for ~ 5 s; if > 3 s = ↓ blood flow to extremities (↓ CO)

3.10   Diaphoresis
Profuse sweating
- Abnormal if seen in the patient who is resting in bed
- Seen in patient who is in shock, hypoxemic or suffers from myocardial infarction (MI)

3.11   Dyspnea
Patient's sensation of shortness of breath (SOB)
- A result of many pulmonary and other disorders that ↑ work of breathing (WOB)
- Severe dyspnea = when walking a few meters or even at rest

Orthopnea
Dyspnea while lying down; suggests CHF ± obstructive lung disease

Platypnea
Dyspnea while sitting up; may suggest R - L intracardiac shunt

Paroxysmal nocturnal dyspnea (PND)
Sudden onset of SOB and orthopnea during sleep; suggests CHF

Differential diagnosis of dyspnea	
Lungs	• Airway: asthma, COPD, fixed narrowing due to tumor, infection • Parenchymal: infection, ILD, pulmonary edema • Pleural: pleural effusion, pneumothorax • Pulm vascular disease: PE, pulm hypertension (PH) • Upper airway obstruction: epiglottitis, croup, foreign body, tracheal stenosis
Cardiovascular	CHF, coronary artery disease (CAD), acute MI, arrhythmias, anemia
Chest wall/ neuromuscular	Spine and rib deformities (eg, kyphoscoliosis), diaphragm/ intercostals muscles, ALS
Psychogenic	Panic attacks, hyperventilation, anxiety, pain
Increased resp. drive	• Hypoxemia: COPD, pneumonia, pleural effusion • Hypercapnia: COPD, kyphoscoliosis • Metabolic acidosis: renal failure • Pregnancy
Abdomen	Results in physical constraint on respiration: ascites, pregnancy, obesity

3.12   Percussion

Resonance
Hollow, low pitch sound produced by normal lungs

Hyperresonance
Booming sound heard with ↑ air in thorax: hyperinflation (asthma, COPD), PTX

Flat
Soft sound heard over airless tissue (muscle, bone): pneumonia, atelectasis, consolidation

Dull
Muffled, thud-like sound heard over areas with little air present

Normal:
Liver, heart

Abnormal:
Atelectasis, pleural effusion, consolidation

Tympany
Loud drum-like sound heard over air filled area

Normal:
Stomach

Abnormal:
Large PTX

3.13   Chest Pain

Pleuritic
Sudden, sharp pain; ↑ on inspiration, cough ± laugh and ↓ with breath hold; may be due to **pleurisy** OR pneumonia, pleural effusion, PTX, pulmonary embolism, tuberculosis

Nonpleuritic
Usually constant and may radiate; may be due to MI, esophagitis, trauma or inflammation of the chest wall (muscles, bones or cartilage)

Differential diagnosis	
Pulmonary	Pleuritis, pneumonia, bronchitis, trauma, lung CA, pneumothorax, PE, pulm. infarct
Cardiac	MI, angina, CHF, arrhythmias, aortic dissection, aortic aneurysm, pericarditis
Thoracic	Trauma, muscle spasm, chest trauma, rib fractures, costochondritis, intercostals myositis
Other	Esophagitis, GI carcinoma, pancreatitis, breast lesions, psychogenic, panic attack

3.14   Sputum Examination

Mucoid (White/clear)

Asthma, COPD, viral pneumonia

Mucopurulent

Yellow + mucoid; chronic bronchitis, acute bacterial infection
(↑ white blood cells [WBC])

Purulent

Yellow or green (fetid odor); bronchiectasis, lung abscess, pneumonia

Brown

Old blood; Klebsiella pneumonia

Red (Bloody)

Bronchiectasis, tuberculosis (TB), lung cancer, pulmonary infarct

Hemoptysis

= Coughing up blood from tracheobronchial tree

Hematemesis

= Blood originating from upper gastrointestinal (GI) tract
(dark, coffee color)

Pink, frothy

Pulmonary edema

3.15   Auscultation

	Description	Cause/comment
Normal breath sounds		
Tracheal/bronchial	Hollow sound heard over trachea/large airways	If over periphery = consolidation
Bronchovesicular	Heard near large airways	If ↓ = consolidation
Vesicular	Airy sound heard over periphery	If ↓ = ↓ local ventilation (pleural effusion, PTX ?)
Abnormal breath sounds		
Crackles	Popping sound	Atelectasis, CHF/ pulmonary edema, fibrosis, pneumonia
Rhonchi	Rattling, bubbling sound; due to air moving through secretions in large airways	Chronic bronchitis, pneumonia, pulmonary edema
Wheeze	Whistling sound as airflow moves through narrowed airways	Asthma, COPD
Pleural rub	Rubbing sound ⇒ inflamed pleura rubbing against each other	Pleurisy, TB, pneumonia
↑ Breath sounds	Consolidation ⇒ fibrosis, pneumonia, atelectasis	
↓ Breath sounds	↓ Airflow (mucus, obstruction), ↑ chest wall thickness (muscle, fat), pleural effusion, hyperinflation (asthma, COPD)	

Expected features in common respiratory disorders

Signs	Pleural fluid, e.g. pleural effusion	Consolidation, e.g. pneumonia	Airway obstruction	Pneumo-thorax	Lung collapse, e.g. atelectasis
Percussion	Dullness	Dullness	Resonant	Hyper-resonant	Dullness
Expansion	↓ on affected side	↓ on affected side	Symmetrical reduction	↓ on affected side	↓ on affected side
Breath sounds	↓ or absent, possibly bronchial	Bronchial, crackles, rhonchi	↓, wheeze, prolonged expiration	↓ or absent	↓ to absent
Vocal fremitus	↓ or absent	Increased	Normal in bronchitis, ↓ in emphysema	↓ to absent	↓ to absent

3.16   Cough

Differential Diagnosis

Pulmonary

Chronic bronchitis, pneumonia, lower respiratory tract infection, TB, asthma, lung abscess, bronchiectasis, cancer, PE, laryngitis, postnasal drip, chronic sinusitis, inhalation of irritant

Other

CHF, mitral stenosis, GERD, esophageal stricture, esophageal-bronchial fistula

3.17   Newborn Assessment

3.17.1   Apgar score

Sign	0	1	2
Respiratory effort	None	Weak	Good, crying
Heart rate	None	< 100	> 100
Reflex irritability (to suctioning)	None	Grimace	Cry, cough, sneeze
Muscle tone	None, limp	Some flexion	Active
Color	Pale, blue	Body pink, extremities blue	Fully pink

Done at 1 min and 5 mins (every 5 mins until score > 7) post-delivery to evaluate if newborn requires immediate resuscitation ± transfer to medical intensive care unit.
Treatment based on score:
≥ 7 = normal: observe, keep warm
4 - 6 = moderate depression: blow-by O_2, bulb suction, warm, tactile stimulation
≤ 3 = severe depression!! Bag-mask ventilation (BMV) 100% O_2, suction, intubate if HR < 100 beats/min and no improvement in ≤ 1 min; if HR < 60 or 60 - 80 beats/min with PPV, compression required

3.17.2   Silverman score

Sign	0	1	2
Upper chest movement	Synchronized	Inspiratory lag	Asynchronous (see-saw)
Lower chest retractions	None	Slight	Marked
Xiphoid retractions	None	Slight	Marked
Nasal flaring	None	Minimal	Marked
Grunting	None	Stethoscope only	Naked ear

Evaluates degree of respiratory distress in newborns (not always done); scoring is **reverse** of Apgar: higher score = higher distress

Score:

0 - 3 = no respiratory distress
4 - 6 = moderate respiratory distress
7 - 10 = severe respiratory distress

3.17.3 Vital signs

Age	Respiratory rate (breaths/min)	Heart rate (beats/min)	Blood pressure (mmHg)
Newborn	30 - 60	120 - 170	70/50 (60 - 80/20 - 60)
6 months	25 - 40	120 - 140	90/60
1 - 3 years	20 - 30	80 - 110	95 - 105/55 -65
4 - 6 years	18 - 25	75 - 110	95 - 110/60 - 70
6 - 8 years	15 - 22	70 - 110	95 - 115/60 - 75
9 - 12 years	15 - 20	70 - 100	110 - 125/60 - 80
> 13 years	12 - 20	60 - 100	100 - 120/60 - 80

Temperature: 36.5 - 37.5°C

Must keep newborn warm (cooling = ↑ VO_2 and at ~ 35°C infant needs 2 x as much as O_2 to survive).

Hypothermia (< 36°C) often a sign of newborn infection.

3.17.4 Signs and symptoms of respiratory distress in the newborn and pediatric patient

Nasal flaring

Infant or child widens nostrils in an attempt to get more air into the lungs, as a result of 'air hunger'

Grunting

Sound heard at end of exhalation. It is a natural physiologic mechanism that creates positive pressure in alveoli in order to counteract ↓ lung volumes (i.e. respiratory distress syndrome [RDS], atelectasis, pneumonia). When the infant exhales against fully or partially closed glottis, this ⇒ pressure back up in alveoli, which ⇒ ↑ FRC and therefore ↑ PaO_2

Retractions
↑ negative intrathoracic pressure causes the space between ribs to be pulled inward. Intercostal, substernal or supraclavicular retractions are a sign of respiratory distress. Retractions are usually due to stiff lungs because the patient must create greater negative pressure to open alveoli. May also be secondary to upper airway obstruction (croup, epiglottitis) or cardiac disease

Tracheal tug
Sucking in of tissue found over sternal notch

Paradoxical or 'see-saw' breathing
May indicate flail chest in children and/or severe respiratory distress. Inspiratory effort draws chest in while abdomen is pushed out

Stridor
High pitched sound heard on inspiration; indicates partial upper airway obstruction (e.g. croup, epiglottitis, postextubation laryngeal edema, vocal cord paralysis)

Wheezing causes
Asthma, bronchiolitis, foreign body obstruction, vocal cord paralysis and mucus plugs

Cyanosis
Bluish discoloration of skin, mucus membranes and nail beds. Noticeable when > 5 g of unsaturated Hb is present. Some causes: hypoxemia due to pulmonary or extrapulmonary R - L shunt, V/Q mismatch (i.e. congenital heart disease, RDS, persistent pulmonary hypertension of the newborn [PPHN])

Acrocyanosis
Peripheral cyanosis (hands and feet) alone is a sign of peripheral vasoconstriction (e.g. circulatory failure) and may not be indicative of hypoxia

Capillary refill
Pinching infant's nail bed for a few seconds and releasing it to see how long it takes for blanched tissue to return to normal color.
If > 3 s, may indicate ↓ CO or hypothermia (vasoconstriction)

Jaundice
If present at birth, it suggests meconium aspiration (especially when yellow cord or nail beds). If after birth, suspect ↑ bilirubin

Scaphoid abdomen

Hollow or flat abdomen which is consistent with diaphragmatic hernia. It results from abdominal contents entering thorax, causing a hollow abdomen

BIBLIOGRAPHY

Des Jardins T, Burton G: Clinical Manifestations and Assessment of Respiratory Disease, 5th ed. Elsevier, 2006.

Czervinske MP, Barnhart SL: Perinatal and Pediatric Respiratory Care, 2nd ed. Saunders, Elsevier Science, 2003.

Hess DR et al: Respiratory Care: Principles and Practice, WB Saunders, 2002.

Wilkins R. et al: Egan's Fundamentals of Respiratory Care, 8th ed. Elsevier Science Limited, 2003.

4. Arterial Blood Gases

4.1 Assessing Oxygenation

4.1.1 Oxygen transport: transported in blood in 2 ways

Dissolved O_2 in blood plasma
- Responsible for PO_2
- Normally insignificant: of ~ 5 ml O_2 used from every 100 ml of blood by tissues, only ~ 3% is dissolved in plasma, accounting for only 3% of O_2 taken by tissues at rest
- At normal PO_2 of 100 mmHg, dissolved O_2 ~ 0.2 ml/dl
- Equation: **dissolved $O_2 = PaO_2 \times 0.003$**
- Things to be considered:
  - Even if PO_2 ~ 600 mmHg (100% O_2), dissolved O_2 is only ~ 2 ml/dl blood = only ~ 35% of O_2 demand at rest
    $P_AO_2 = (760 - 47) \times 1 - P_ACO_2 = 673 \times 0.003$ ~ 2 ml/dl
  - At 3 atm (2280 mmHg) + 100% O_2 by hyperbaric chamber, dissolved O_2 ~ 6 ml/dl, which can sustain life; dissolved $O_2 = (2280 - 47) - 40 = 2180 \times 0.003 = 6.5$ ml/dl

O_2 bound to Hb
- Most of O_2 (~ 98%) is carried by Hb, an intra-erythrocyte protein molecule with 4 iron atoms, to which up to 4 O_2 molecules combine reversibly
- Hb also carries CO_2, but not at same binding site: O_2 binds to heme while CO_2 binds to globin

Oxyhemoglobin (HbO_2):
Hb bound to O_2

Deoxyhemoglobin:
Hb not bound to O_2

Myoglobin (Mb):
Muscle protein serving as O_2 reserve and facilitates O_2 movement within skeletal and heart muscle. Each Mb molecule binds 1 O_2 molecule.

4.1.2   Oxygenation parameters

Arterial oxygen tension, PaO_2
- Dissolved O_2 (O_2 tension in plasma)
- Does NOT guarantee adequate tissue oxygenation because it is only 1 factor in oxygen transport
- Also, hypoxemia ≠ automatic tissue hypoxia, but = possibility

NOTE: When Hb is unable to carry O_2 (CO poisoning), high FIO_2 is given to ↑ amount of dissolved O_2 (PaO_2), but patient may be severely hypoxic despite ↑/normal PaO_2 (must check SaO_2, HbCO, CaO_2).

- **Normal value:** (PaO_2 is based on age, FIO_2, Pb, $PaCO_2$)
          Predicted PaO_2 = 110 - ½ age, at sea level, 21% O_2:
          70 - 100 mmHg
          Newborn: 40 - 70 mmHg
          60 y: ≥ 80 mmHg
          70 y: ≥ 70 mmHg
          80 y: ≥ 60 mmHg
          90 y: ≥ 50 mmHg
          Chronic hypoxemia (COPD): 50 - 60 mmHg
          [also $PaCO_2$ ~ 50 - 60 mmHg]
- ↑ **with:** hyperventilation, ↑ FIO_2
- ↓ **with:** ↓FIO_2, hypoxemia (V/Q mismatch, shunt, ↓ Pb, diffusion defect)

Hypoxemia	PaO_2
Mild	< 80 mmHg
Moderate	< 60 mmHg
Severe	< 40 mmHg

PaO_2 is less important than SaO_2 and CaO_2 as an evaluator of adequate oxygenation.

Arterial oxygen saturation, SaO_2
- Determined mainly by PaO_2

NOTE: Hb gives up only ~ 25% of O_2 to tissues (SvO_2 of 75% and PvO_2 of 40 mmHg); this serves as a reserve O_2 supply during ↑ demand.

- NOT a measure of O_2 or Hb concentration, so:
100% Hb saturation (and normal PaO_2) ≠ automatic normal CaO_2
(e.g. ↓ Hb in anemia = ↓ CaO_2, but SaO_2 can be 100%)

Low SaO_2 ≠ automatic low CaO_2, as Hb could increase
• Normal value: 95 - 98% (chronic hypoxemia [e.g. COPD]: 85 - 90%)

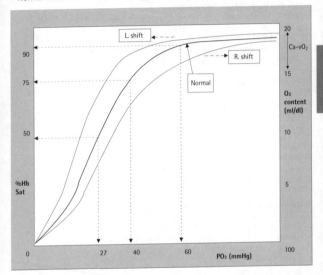

Fig. 6 Oxyhemoglobin dissociation curve

Factors that shift oxyhemoglobin curve

Left shift: ↓ P50 = ↑ O_2 affinity for Hb	Right shift: ↑ P50 = ↓ O_2 affinity for Hb
• ↓ Temperature	• ↑ Temperature
• ↓ $PaCO_2$, ↑ pH (alkalosis)	• ↑ $PaCO_2$, ↓ pH (acidosis)
• COHb	• ↑ 2,3 DPG
• ↓ 2,3 DPG (stored blood)	(chronic hypoxemia, ↑ altitude)
• fetHb	• abnormal Hb (sickle cell)

P50: PO_2 at which Hb is 50% saturated; normally 27 mmHg; measure of Hb affinity for O_2

Upper flat part (PaO_2 > 60 mmHg):
large PaO_2 change (from 60 to 100 mmHg) = small SaO_2 change (90 - 97%); and small CaO_2 change

Steep part (PaO_2 < 60 mmHg):
small PaO_2 change = large SaO_2 and CaO_2 change; PO_2 ↓ from 60 to 20 mmHg = SaO_2 ↓ from 90% to 30%. Therefore, SaO_2 of 90% is critical

Total oxygen content

Arterial:
- CaO_2 = (O_2 combined with Hb) + (dissolved O_2 in plasma)
  = (Hb x 1.34 x SaO_2) + (PaO_2 x 0.003)
- With normal Hb of 15 g, PaO_2 of 100 mmHg and SaO_2 of 97%, normal CaO_2 ~ 20 ml/dl
- Normal value: 18 - 21 ml/dl

Mixed venous:
- CvO_2 = (Hb x 1.34 x SvO_2) + (PvO_2 x 0.003)
- Indicates O_2 left in the blood after leaving tissues
- Normal value: 12 - 15 ml/dl

Arterio–mixed venous O_2 content difference, C(a – v)O_2

C(a – v)O_2 = CaO_2 – CvO_2 = 20 – 15 = 5 ml/dl
- A measure of O_2 extracted by the tissues (~25%)
- ↑ **with:** ↓ CO, ↑ VO_2 (exercise, seizures, hyperthermia)
- ↓ **with:** ↑ CO, sepsis, cyanide poison, hypothermia
- Normal value: 4 - 5 ml/dl

Oxygen delivery, DO_2

DO_2 = (CaO_2 x CO) x 10 = (20 x 5) x 10 = 1000 ml/min
- ↑ **with:** ↑ blood oxygenation, ↑ CO, ↑ Hb
- ↓ **with:** ↓ blood oxygenation, ↓ CO, ↓ Hb
- Normal value: 800 - 1000 ml/min

Oxygen consumption, VO_2

VO_2 = CO x (CaO_2 – CvO_2) x 10
- Normally, 250 ml/min of 1000 ml/min O_2 available is extracted by the tissues, leaving mixed venous blood ~ 75% saturated. This serves as O_2 reserve in cases of stress

- ↑ **with:** exercise, hyperthermia, seizures, ↑ metabolism
- ↓ **with:** hypothermia, cyanide poison, ↓ CO, ↓ metabolism
- Normal value:
  - 250 ml/min
  - 125 - 165 $ml/min/m^2$ when related to body surface area (BSA) VO_2/BSA

Oxygen extraction ratio, O_2ER

$O_2ER = C(a - v)O_2 \div CaO_2 = 5$ ml/dl $\div$ 20 ml/dl = 0.25 (25%)
- ↑ **with:** ↓ CO, ↑ VO_2 (exercise, seizures, hyperthermia), anemia
- ↓ **with:** ↑ CO, sepsis, cyanide poison, ↑ Hb, hypothermia
- Tissues normally extract 25% of CaO_2 (range: 20 - 30%).

Mixed venous oxygen tension, PvO_2

- Best index of tissue oxygenation
- < 30 mmHg = ↑ risk of tissue hypoxia
- Normal range: 35 - 45 mmHg

Mixed venous oxygen saturation, SvO_2

- < 35% indicates inadequate tissue oxygenation
- ↑ **with:** ↑ CO, sepsis, cyanide poison, hypothermia
- ↓ **with:** ↓ CO, ↑ VO_2 (exercise, seizures, hyperthermia)
- Normal value: 70 - 75%

Alveolar – arterial oxygen tension difference, $P_A - aO_2$

$P_A - aO_2 = P_AO_2 - PaO_2$ [A – a gradient]
- Distinguishes shunt from V/Q mismatch
- Normal value:
  - Room air: 5 - 20 mmHg
  - 100% O_2: 25 - 65 mmHg

Arterial – alveolar oxygen tension ratio, PaO_2/PAO_2

PaO_2/PAO_2 (a - A ratio)
- Normal value:
  - 0.8 - 0.9
  - 0.75 in elderly
- Abnormal: < 0.6

Arterial oxygen tension to FIO_2 ratio, PaO_2/FIO_2 (P/F ratio)

- Normal Values: > 300
- Abnormal: < 300
- Acute RDS (ARDS): < 200

Pulmonary shunt, Qs/Qt

$Qs/Qt = (CcO_2 - CaO_2)/(CcO_2 - CvO_2)$

- Normal value: 2 - 5%
- < 10% shunt: normal
- 10 - 20% shunt = intrapulmonary abnormality (usually insignificant)
- 20 - 30% shunt = significant shunt
- > 30% shunt = life threatening

Alveolar oxygen tension, P_AO_2

$P_AO_2 = (Pb - PH_2O) \times FIO_2 - PaCO_2 \times 1.25$

- Estimated: $P_AO_2 = 150 - PaCO_2$
- Normal value: 100 - 105 mmHg on room air and 660 mmHg on 100% O_2

Hemoglobin, Hb

- Oxyhemoglobin: 93 - 100%
- Carboxyhemoglobin: < 2%, < 5% in smokers
- Methemoglobin: < 2%
- Normal range:
  - M: 14 - 18 g/dl
  - F: 12 - 16 g/dl

4.1.3   Causes and types of hypoxia

Category/Causes	PaO_2	SaO_2	CaO_2	↑ FIO_2 helps?
1. Hypoxemic hypoxia				
↓ PIO_2 : due to ↑ altitude (↓ Pb) = ↓ PaO_2	↓	↓	↓	yes
Hypoventilation: ↓ V_A = ↓ P_AO_2 = ↑ P_ACO_2	↓	↓	↓	yes
V/Q mismatch: most common cause	↓	↓	↓	yes
R – L shunt: ARDS, pneumonia, atelectasis	↓	↓	↓	**no**
Diffusion defect: rare - severe ILD?	↓	↓	↓	yes

2. Anemic hypoxia				
Anemia: mild anemia of Hb ~ 10 g usually not of concern because of compensation by: (a) O_2ER is ~ 25% = large O_2 reserve; (b) ↑CO: severe anemia of Hb < 6 - 7 g is of concern as compensatory mechanism is overloaded	N	N	↓	**no**
Carbon monoxide poisoning: ↓ functioning Hb due to formation of COHb	N	↓ SpO_2 may be falsely normal	↓	yes
3. Circulatory (hypoperfusion) hypoxia				
Due to ↓ blood flow to tissues (↓ CO) or hypovolemia (shock, hemorrhage)	N	N	N	poor
4. Histotoxic hypoxia				
Tissue unable to use O_2: cyanide poison; O_2 not extracted = ↑ PvO_2	N	N	N	poor

Key: N = normal; ↑ = increased; ↓ = decreased

Relationship between PaO_2 and SaO_2% (assumes Hb of 15 g)	
PaO_2	**SaO_2**
27	50
30	57
40	**75**
50	84
60	**90**
80	95
90	97
100	**98**
150	99
250	**100**
600 (100% O_2)	100
Rule of thumb: $FIO_2 \times 5 = PaO_2$ (estimated)	

4.2   Assessing Ventilation

4.2.1   Carbon dioxide transport: transported in 3 different ways

$PaCO_2$ is the best indicator of adequate ventilation

Dissolved CO_2
- ~ 5 - 10% is carried in plasma
- It combines with water to form carbonic acid: ($CO_2 + H_2O \Rightarrow H_2CO_3$)

Carbaminohemoglobin
- ~ 5 - 10% is bound to Hb as carbamino

Bicarbonate (HCO_3^-)
- ~ 80 - 90% transported as bicarbonate
- In RBC, carbonic acid rapidly undergoes hydration due to carbonic anhydrase (CA) enzyme, to form H^+ and HCO_3^- ions [$CO_2 + H_2O \overset{CA}{\rightleftharpoons} H_2CO_3 \Rightarrow HCO_3^- + H^+$]

Acid - base disturbances		PO₂ (mmHg)	SO₂ (%)	PCO₂ (mmHg)	pH	HCO₃⁻ (mEq/l)
Normal blood gas values	Arterial	80 - 100	93 - 98	35 - 45	7.35 - 7.45	22 - 26
	Venous	35 - 45	65 - 75	40 - 50	7.31 - 7.41	22 - 26
Respiratory acidosis				↑	↓	N (↑)
Respiratory alkalosis				↓	↑	N (↓)
Metabolic acidosis				N (↓)	↓	↓
Metabolic alkalosis				N (↑)	↑	↑

Bold arrow = primary change
Thin arrow = secondary change
Arrow in brackets = compensation
N = normal

4.2.2 Newborn blood gas values

	PO$_2$ (mmHg)	pH	PCO$_2$ (mmHg)	HCO$_3$⁻ (mEq/l)
Newborn: birth	< 60	7.2 - 7.3	45 - 55	20 - 24
1 hour	60 - 70	7.3 - 7.35	40 - 55	18 - 22
1 day	80 - 100	7.3 - 7.4	30 - 40	20 - 22
Umbilical artery	7 - 23	7.1 - 7.4	35 - 60	14 - 21
Umbilical vein	15 - 40	7.15 - 7.4	30 - 55	12 - 23

4.2.3 Quick approach to interpreting arterial blood gas measurements (ABGs)

STEP 1: categorize pH
|

Check pH: normal 7.35 - 7.45
pH < 7.35 = acidosis
pH > 7.45 = alkalosis

|

STEP 2: determine primary disturbance (2 arrows)
|

A. Check PaCO$_2$: normal 35 - 45 mmHg (up to 55 - 60 mmHg in CO$_2$ retainers) B. Check HCO$_3$⁻: normal 22 - 26 mEq/L				
Compensation = 1 arrow	pH	PaCO$_2$	HCO$_3$⁻	Go to
Respiratory acidosis	↓	↑↑	↑	Step 3A
Respiratory alkalosis	↑	↓↓	↓	Step 3A
Metabolic acidosis	↓	↓	↓↓	Step 3B
Metabolic alkalosis	↑	↑	↑↑	Step 3B

|

STEP 3: determine compensation (acute or chronic)

Primary disorder	Secondary response	Time to full compensation
A. Check for metabolic compensation in primary respiratory disturbance		
Respiratory acidosis	acute: ↑ HCO_3^- of 1 mEq/L/ ↑ 10 mmHg $PaCO_2$	5 - 10 min
	chronic: ↑ HCO_3^- of 3 mEq/L/ ↑ 10 mmHg $PaCO_2$	72 - 96 h
Respiratory alkalosis	acute: ↓ HCO_3^- of 2 mEq/L/ ↓ 10 mmHg $PaCO_2$	5 - 10 min
	chronic: ↓ HCO_3^- of 5 mEq/L/ ↓ 10 mmHg $PaCO_2$	48 - 72 h
B. Check for respiratory compensation in primary metabolic disturbance		
Metabolic acidosis	↓ $PaCO_2$ of 1 - 1.3 mmHg for 1 mEq/L ↓ HCO_3^-	12 - 24 h
Metabolic alkalosis	↑ $PaCO_2$ of 0.4 - 0.7 mmHg for 1 mEq/L ↑ HCO_3^-	24 - 36 h

STEP 4: determine anion gap (AG) vs non-AG metabolic acidosis (if present)

Calculate AG: from routine serum assay

- Helpful in narrowing down potential causes of metabolic acidosis
- Normal AG = 12 mEq/L
- AG = Na^+ - (Cl^- + HCO_3^-)
- AG metabolic acidosis = AG > 12
- Non-AG metabolic acidosis = AG < 12

4.2.4 Some causes of acid – base disorders:

Respiratory acidosis (hypoventilation)

- CNS depression: cerebrovascular accident (CVA), sedatives, lesions/tumors, obesity hypoventilation syndrome
- Neuromuscular: amyotrophic lateral sclerosis (ALS), Guillain-Barré syndrome, myasthenia gravis, polio
- Lung disease: COPD, pneumonia
- Airway obstruction: sleep apnea, foreign objects, bronchospasm
- Chest wall: severe kyphoscoliosis, chest trauma, inadequate mechanical ventilation

Respiratory alkalosis (hyperventilation)

- CNS disorders: CVA, drugs (salicylates, progesterone), anxiety, trauma, encephalitis
- Hypoxemia (most common cause)
- Parenchymal lung disease: pneumonia, ILD, asthma, pulmonary edema
- Metabolic: sepsis, fever, hyperthyroidism, bacteremia, hepatic failure/coma

Metabolic acidosis

Anion-gap acidosis:	Non-Ag acidosis:
MUDPILES (mnemonic)	**ACCRUED (mnemonic)**
- **M**ethanol	- **A**cid infusion: HCl, NH_4Cl
- **U**remia	- **C**ompensation for respiratory alkalosis
- **D**iabetic ketoacidosis	- **C**arbonic anhydrase inhibitor: Diamox
- **P**araldehyde	- **R**enal tubular acidosis
- **I**ron or isoniazid	- **U**reteral diversion
- **L**actic acidosis	- **E**xtra alimentation or hyperalimentation
- **E**thylene glycol (antifreeze)	- **D**iarrhea: GI loss of HCO_3^-
- **S**alicylates	

Metabolic alkalosis

- Vomiting
- Alkali ingestion: HCO_3^- during arrest
- Hypokalemia
- Hypochloremia: nasogastric (NG) suctioning
- Aldosteronism (Cushing's syndrome)
- Overdiuresis
- Excess gluco- or mineralocorticoids

4.3   Noninvasive Monitoring of Blood Gases

4.3.1   Pulse oximetry

Quick noninvasive estimation of O_2 saturation of Hb in arterial blood
• Abbreviated SpO_2
• Accuracy: ± 3% for saturations > 70%; therefore, an SpO_2 of 90% may correspond to co-oximetry measurement of ~ 87 - 93%

Indications
• Need for oxygenation monitoring of FIO_2
• Special procedures: intubation, bronchoscopy, catheterization, sleep apnea monitoring
• Probe usually placed on finger or toe; also over ear lobe/nasal bridge

Accuracy is affected by
• Motion artifact
• Dark nail polish = ↓ reading
• COHb = false high SpO_2 because COHb is read as oxyhemoglobin
• Low perfusion
• Intravascular dyes (methylene blue) = false low SpO_2
• Ambient light

4.3.2   Capnography (End-tidal CO_2; $ETCO_2$)

$ETCO_2$

= P_ACO_2 at end of exhalation. It is normally 4.5 - 5.5%, which is equivalent to $PaCO_2$ of 35 - 45 mmHg. It is measured by placing sensor between the endotracheal tube (ETT) and wye adaptor of patient's breathing circuit.

Normal **$ETCO_2$** is usually 2 - 5 mmHg < $PaCO_2$

Difference between **$ETCO_2$** and **$PaCO_2$**:

(1) Dead space ventilation ⇒ ↑ $ETCO_2$ - $PaCO_2$ difference (causes of dead space ventilation: high V_T, pulmonary embolism, ↓ blood flow in pulmonary circulation, hypotension)
(2) Shunting ⇒ ↓ $ETCO_2$ - $PaCO_2$ difference
(causes of shunt: atelectasis, mucus plugs, severe pneumonia)

Causes of ↑ **ETCO$_2$**: ↓ **V/Q**

(1) ↑ VCO$_2$: fever, seizures, sepsis
(2) ↓ V$_A$: COPD, CNS depression (drug OD), leaks in the breathing circuit

Causes of ↓ **ETCO$_2$**: ↑ **V/Q**

(1) ↓ VCO$_2$: pulmonary embolism (PE), pulmon. hypoperfusion, hypothermia
(2) ↑ alveolar ventilation (V$_A$), cardiac arrest, ventilator disconnects, ETT cuff leak

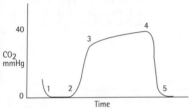

Fig. 7 Normal capnogram or CO$_2$ waveform

1 - 2: Exhalation of dead space gas containing no CO$_2$
2 - 3: Rapid rise of CO$_2$ because alveolar gas is exhaled
        (combination of dead space and alveolar gas)
3 - 4: Exhalation of mostly alveolar gas (alveolar gas plateau)
    4: End-tidal CO$_2$ concentration
4 - 5: Inspiration and rapid fall in CO$_2$

Detection of ventilation problems

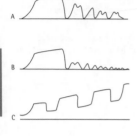

A: Partial airway obstruction or system leak

B: Sudden loss of waveform: airway disconnected, obstructed ETT (plug), kinked tube or cardiac arrest

C: Rebreathing of CO_2: excessive mechanical dead space, inadequate inspiratory gas flow, inadequate expiratory time or hypoventilation

D: Uneven alveolar emptying due to airflow obstruction (COPD, asthma); failure to achieve plateau.

Fig. 8 Pathological capnograms

BIBLIOGRAPHY

Malley WJ: Clinical Blood Gases: Assessment and Intervention, Elsevier Saunders, 2005.

Martin L: All You Really Need to Know to Intepret Arterial Blood Gases, 2nd ed. LWW, 1999.

Shapiro B et al: Clinical Applications of Blood Gases, 5th ed. Mosby, 1994.

5.   Thoracic Imaging

5.1   Chest X-ray (CXR) Interpretation

5.1.1   Terminology

Air bronchogram
Air filled bronchi (appear dark) surrounded by white area (opacity) produced by consolidation or infiltrates

Cavity
Radiolucent area surrounded by radiopaque area (suggests lung abscess)

Consolidation
Solidification (opacification) of the lung tissue such as occurs with pneumonia (alveolar filling)

Diffuse
Spread out (i.e. pneumonia, atelectasis)

Honeycombing
Coarse reticular (net-like) density often seen in pneumoconiosis

Infiltration
Poorly defined radiopaque area (e.g. atelectasis)

Radiopaque
White area (opacity) - organs, fluid

Radiolucent
Dark pattern; lungs inflated with air; ↑ with COPD, asthma

Silhouette sign
Loss of distinction of a common border such as when densities occur next to each other (e.g. pneumonia involving heart border)

5.1.2   Standard X-ray positions

Posteroanterior (PA)
Most commonly used view. Taken with patient upright, max. inspiration (diaphragm ~ 9 - 11th rib posteriorly) and scapulae rotated away from lung fields

Anteroposterior (AP)

Used often for bedridden patients (e.g. ICU) = portable X-ray; heart size is artificially magnified by ~ 20% as a result of the heart being further away from the film; therefore, quality of film is inferior to PA view

Lateral

Allows visualization of lung fields and lung parenchyma behind the heart (patient's arms raised). It supplements PA film

Lateral decubitus

Taken with patient lying on affected side. Used to diagnose/detect suspected pleural effusion

Lordotic

Provides better view of lung apex and right middle lobe. May help detect chronic TB disease

Lateral neck X-ray

Useful in diagnosis of croup (subglottic edema) and epiglottitis (swollen epiglottis - supraglottic)

5.1.3 Systematic approach to CXR interpretation

NOTE: Use systematic approach when interpreting CXR in order to avoid overlooking significant details. Precise order is less important than consistency with which one applies the method.

Position

Spinous processes should be midline in tracheal air column; any slight rotation distorts the view of midline structures and may result in inaccurate interpretation

Soft tissue

If female, identify breast shadows: superimposed over lower lobes (do not confuse with abnormality); 1 breast absent = ↑ hyperlucency over lower lung on affected side. Also, check for subcutaneous air

Bones

Look for fractures, arthritic changes, prior surgery (rib notching)

NOTE: Kyphoscoliosis = more difficult interpretation.

Diaphragm

Right hemidiaphragm is ~ 2 cm higher than left. Costophrenic angles should be clear (> 300 ml fluid can be detected on PA chest). Flat diaphragm = hyperinflation (air trapping, COPD); elevated diaphragm = paralysis, atelectasis, PTX

Heart

Should be < ½ chest width in adults and ≤ 60% in newborns (cardiothoracic ratio does not apply for AP films, as heart is magnified); if > ½ = CHF, cor pulmonale (COPD)

Trachea and mediastinum

Will shift to affected side with atelectasis, fibrosis. Shifts away from affected side with PTX, pleural effusion

Hilum

L. hilum ~ 2 cm higher than R. hilum = main bronchi and central pulmonary vessels (where trachea divides). Enlargement = enlarged lymph nodes?, ↑ PVR?

Lung fields: selected CXR abnormalities	
Atelectasis	↓ volume and elevated hemidiaphragm on affected side; mediastinal shift to affected side; ↑ opacity; scattered densities; air bronchograms
ARDS/Infant respiratory distress syndrome (IRDS)	Diffuse b/l infiltrates; air bronchograms; ↑ opacity (white-out secondary to ↓ aeration due to atelectasis; volume loss; 'ground glass' (reticulogranular pattern) - honeycomb pattern (small cystic areas)
Bronchiectasis	Best seen on computed tomography (CT) scan with 1 - 2 mm slices; on CXR shows as tubular shadows (tram tracks); results from repeated bronchial infections - scarring
Bronchopulmonary dysplasia (BPD)	Newborn disease - hyperaeration with cystic areas
COPD	↑ AP diameter; depressed diaphragm; ↑ retrosternal airspaces on lateral film; ↑ radiolucency (hyperinflation); heart may appear small (but is not), as lungs are bigger as a result of overinflation

Congenital diaphragmatic hernia (CDH)	Newborn disease - stomach contents in thorax due to diaphragm malformation. May see NG tube enter abdomen and pass back up to chest area
CHF	↑ vascular markings; cardiomegaly; Kerley B-lines ~ 1 mm thick and 1 - 2 cm long: = thickened interlobular septa due to pulmonary edema
Croup	Pediatric disease - lateral neck X-ray shows haziness in subglottic area
Epiglottitis	Pediatric disease - lateral neck X-ray shows supraglottic haziness
Fibrosis, pulmonary	↑ peripheral markings; 'ground glass' appearance (reticulonodular infiltrates); honeycombing
Lung abscess	Fluid-filled cavity resulting in ↑ opacity
Meconium aspiration syndrome (MAS)	Newborn - if severe, b/l infiltrates and air trapping
Pleural effusion	Blunting of costophrenic angle - white out (↑ opacity) on affected side
Pneumonia	↑ opacity ± air bronchograms; homogeneous or nonhomogeneous 'fluffy' opacities
Pneumothorax	Dark air space without peripheral lung markings. Results in ↑ radiolucency. With tension PTX: depressed diaphragm on affected side and trachea/mediastinum shift away from affected side
Pulmonary edema	↑ radiopacity; fluffy 'butterfly shape' infiltrates; air bronchograms; possibly cardiomegaly; Kerley-B lines (full lymphatics)
Transient tachypnea of the newborn (TTNB)	Newborn - resembles hyaline membrane disease; distinguishable, in that it clears in ~ 24 h
Position of tubes and catheters	
ETT	Tip should be ~ 2 - 3 cm above carina and ~ 3 cm below vocal cords in adults
Central venous catheter tip	Should be in superior vena cava (SVC), just before right atrium (RA)

Pulmonary artery catheter tip	Should be located in right or left pulmonary artery, ~ 5 cm distal to main bifurcation of pulmonary artery (PA)
Intra-aortic balloon pump (IABP) catheter tip	Should be just distal to subclavian artery
Tracheostomy tube (TT) tip	Should be ~ $\frac{1}{2}$ - $\frac{1}{3}$ of distance between stoma and carina
Umbilical artery catheter (UAC)	In neonates should be positioned between 7th - 8th (T7 - T8) or 3rd - 4th (L3 - L4) vertebra

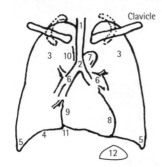

Fig. 9 CXR interpretation, a.p.

1. Trachea
2. Carina
3. Lung fields
4. Dome of diaphragm
5. Costophrenic angle

6. Hilum
7. Aortic arch
8. Left heart border
9. Right heart border

10. Superior vena cava
11. Inferior vena cava
12. Stomach gas bubble

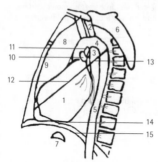

Fig. 10 CXR interpretation, transverse

1. Heart
2. Trachea
3. Pulmonary trunk and hilum
4. Arch of aorta
5. Descending aorta
6. Scapula
7. Stomach gas bubble
8. Anterior space

9. Sternum
10. Right pulmonary artery
11. Left pulmonary artery
12. Oblique fissure
13. Horizontal fissure
14. Right hemidiaphragm
15. Left hemidiaphragm

5.2   Other Imaging Techniques of the Thorax

5.2.1. Computed Tomography (CT)

- Provides a detailed cross-sectional view of the thorax (5 - 10 mm thin slices)
- **High resolution CT (HRCT)** refers to using 1 - 2 mm slice thickness. HRCT is valuable in assessment of diffuse lung parenchymal disease and its major indications include:
  - Evaluation of suspected ILD when CXR is normal or nonspecific
  - Characterization of ILD or solitary pulmonary nodules
  - Diagnosis of bronchiectasis (CT has replaced bronchography as the 'gold standard' diagnostic test for bronchiectasis)

- **Indications for CT:**
  - Detecting and/or confirming presence of mediastinal mass and its size
  - Differentiating pleural from parenchymal masses/abnormalities
  - Detecting pulmonary nodules and subpleural lesions not visible on standard X-ray
  - Staging lung cancer
  - Lung parenchyma and ILD
  - Detecting pulmonary embolism, high specifity, with helical CT scanning conitnously improving sensitivity
  - Can also be used for guidance of needle placement during procedures such as needle biopsy of pulmonary or mediastinal lesions

- **CT features of lung disease:**

○ Nodular pattern	Hypersensitivity pneumonitis, silicosis, asbestosis, metastatic cancer, cryptogenic organizing pneumonia (COP), alveolar microlithiasis, pulmonary hemorrhage
○ Reticular (linear) pattern	Usual interstitial pneumonia (UIP), asbestosis, collagen vascular disease, ILD, pulmonary edema, pulmonary hemorrhage
○ Ground-glass pattern	ARDS/pulmonary edema, PCP, hypersensitivity pneumonitis, sarcoidosis, drug or radiation injury, pulmonary alveolar proteinosis, desquamative interstitial pneumonia (DIP), pulmonary hemorrhage
○ Cysts	Lymphangiomyomatosis (LAM), lymphoid interstitial pneumonia (LIP), pulmonary histiocytosis X, PCP, end-stage UIP
○ Honeycombing (cluster/row of cysts)	[Note: distinguish from emphysema] Usual interstitial pneumonitis (UIP), asbestosis, collagen vascular disease, sarcoidosis, hypersensitivity pneumonitis
○ Consolidation	Organizing pneumonia (OP), pulmonary alveolar proteinosis, eosinophilic pneumonia, lipoid pneumonia, pulmonary edema
○ Mosaic pattern	Embolism, hypersensitivity pneumonitis

- **Spiral (helical) scanning:** Continuous scanning while table with patient moves into CT gantry. Advantage: produces contiguous scanning ⇒ ↓ chance of missing small pulmonary nodules/abnormalities
- Newer technologies allow complete thorax scanning with a single breath-hold

5.2.2. Magnetic Resonance Imaging (MRI)

- Most of indications for thoracic MRI are related to hilar/mediastinal and chest wall abnormalities. Clinical situations where MRI may be useful include:
  - Aortic dissection or aneurysm
  - Hilar, mediastinal and chest wall abnormalities:
    congenital heart disease, tumors, vascular pathology
  - Complicated pleural and diaphragmatic diseases
- **Contraindications:** patients with cardiac pacemakers

5.2.3. Pulmonary Angiography

- Definitive diagnostic technique to detect pulmonary embolism
- Gold standard for confirming the presence of pulmonary arterio-venous malformation; necessary before planning embolization therapy

5.2.4. Ultrasonography (US)

- US has limited use in pulmonary disease. Doppler (duplex) US is the noninvasive technique of choice for detection of deep vein thrombosis (DVT) in lower extremities
- May be helpful in:
  - Assessing/detecting free fluid and localized pockets of loculated fluid in pleural densities
  - Guidance of thoracentesis (e.g. when 'blind' thoracentesis fails)
  - ± Guidance for needle aspiration biopsy of certain pulm. and mediast. lesions

5.2.5. Positron Emission Tomography (PET)

- PET utilizes fluorinated analogue of glucose (FDG) and gives images of lung that highlight areas of increased glucose metabolism. **Malignant cells** have ↑ glucose uptake compared with normal tissues or benign process and appear as ↑ densities on PET images
- Indications:
  - Distinguishing benign and malignant focal pulmonary abnormalities: solitary pulmonary nodules, staging lung cancer
  - Distinguishing fibrosis from tumor in patient treated for lung cancer

5.2.6. Ventilation – Perfusion (V/Q) Scanning: nuclear medicine

- Most commonly performed in detecting and diagnosing **pulmonary embolism**. Lodgement of embolus within a lobar or segmental pulmonary artery ⇒ ↓ or full absence of perfusion in involved region. Ventilation in same area is often maintained, at least for 24 - 48 h
- **Perfusion scintigraph:**
  - Pulmonary perfusion via pulmonary artery can be determined from images (gamma camera) following IV injection of radioactive marker **technetium-99m**
  - Scanning device passes over thorax with gamma radiation providing recorded image of distribution and volume of lung perfusion
- **Ventilation scintigraph:**
  - Measured by scanning the thorax while patient inhales (via specialized rebreathing apparatus) radioactive gas **xenon**
  - Radioactivity equilibration of all lung regions takes ~ 3 - 5 min

BIBLIOGRAPHY

Farrell MA et al: Imaging the Thorax. In, Hess DR et al: Respiratory Care: Principles and Practice, WB Saunders, 2002.

Hansell DM, Padley SPG: Imaging. In, Albert RK, Spiro SS, Jett JR (eds): Clinical Respiratory Medicine, 2nd ed. Mosby 2004.

Lynch DA, Menon P: Imaging of Lung Disease. In, Crapo JD et al (eds): Baum's Textbook of Pulmonary Diseases, 7th ed. LWW, 2004.

6.   Pulmonary Function Tests (PFT)

6.1   Indications, Contraindications

Indications for PFT

- To evaluate for presence of lung disease
- To assess severity and progression of known lung disease
- To diagnose/differentiate obstructive vs restrictive lung disease
- To assess the effectiveness of therapy
- To evaluate the amount of disability
- To assess postoperative complications

Contraindications

- Poor coordination or unable to perform (very old or very young)
- Contagious disease (e.g. TB)
- Pneumothorax
- Aneurysms
- Hernias
- Angina or recent MI
- Recent eye, abdominal or thoracic surgery

6.2   Spirometry

Volumes	Max. inspiration	Capacities		
		IC	VC	TLC
IRV				
VT				
ERV		FRC		
	Max. expiration			
RV			RV	

Fig. 11 Normal Spirogramm

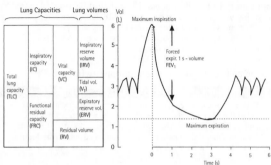

Fig. 12 FEV$_1$

6.2.1   Measuring FRC, RV and TLC

Because RV cannot be exhaled, it cannot be measured by spirometry.
Thus, FRC is measured by non-spirometric methods (He-dilution, N$_2$-washout,
or plethysmography) from which the RV and TLC can be calculated.

RV = FRC - ERV

TLC = FRC + RV

Helium dilution (closed circuit)
- Patient breathes a gas mixture of 10% He, 21% O$_2$, rest N$_2$ until equilibration
  occurs, at which point FRC is calculated
- Takes ~ 7 min, if > 7 min = obstruction

Nitrogen washout (open circuit)
- Patient inhales 100% O$_2$ for ~ 7 min until N$_2$ is washed out from lungs to ≤ 1%
- If > 7 min = obstructive lung disease

Plethysmography (body box)
- Patient pants against occluded mouthpiece while pressures and volumes are
  obtained

- Uses Boyle's law to get total thoracic gas volume (TGV) at FRC even if distal to obstructed airways. Measures trapped gas also, unlike He-dilution and N_2-washout methods, which measure only volume in communicating airways
- Therefore, FRC, RV and TLC values obtained with body box are > values obtained with He-dilution or N_2-washout techniques

6.2.2 Common tests obtained from spirometry (from FVC)

	Expiratory Flows	Interpretation
FVC	**Forced vital capacity:** maximum volume of gas exhaled as forcefully and rapidly as possible after maximally inhaling. From FVC important measurements include FEV_1, $FEF_{25-75\%}$ and PEF	• Normally exhaled in 4 - 6 s • COPD patients may need ≥ 8 - 15 s to exhale (F)VC • ↓ FVC in both obstructive and restrictive lung diseases
FEV_1	**Forced expiratory volume in 1s:** volume exhaled in the first second of FVC maneuver. Often expressed as percent of FVC (FEV_1/FVC ratio or $FEV_{1\%}$). Decreases ~ 30 ml/year after age 30, but in COPD patients this decrease is 2 - 4 times larger (60 - 120 ml/year)	**Normal:** $\geq 80\%$, $\geq 70\%$ acceptable in elderly **Obstruction:** ($\downarrow FEV_1$, $\downarrow FEV_1$/FVC) • mild: 60 - 80% of predicted • moderate: 40 - 60% predicted • severe: < 40% predicted **Restriction:** ($\downarrow$ FEV1, norm/$\uparrow$ FEV_1/FVC)
$FEV_{25-75\%}$	**Forced expiratory flow between 25% and 75% of FVC:** average flow during middle portion of FVC. Reflects status of small - medium sized airways. Highly variable test	**Normal:** 3.5 - 5 L/s (210 - 300 L/min) $\downarrow$ $FEF_{25-75\%}$: may indicate early stages of small airway disease Norm/$\downarrow$ $FEF_{25-75\%}$: restriction
$FEF_{200-1200}$	**Forced expiratory flow 200 - 1200 ml:** average flow between 200 and 1200 ml of FVC. Reflects integrity of large airways	**Normal:** 5.5 - 8 L/s (330 - 480 L/min) $\downarrow$ $FEF_{200-1200}$: large airway obstruction restrictive lung disorders

| PEF | **Peak expiratory flow:** maximal flow during FVC. Usually measured with cheap portable peak flow meters to evaluate day-to-day degree of bronchospasm in asthma patients | **Normal:**
M: 500 - 600 L/min (8 -10 L/s)
F: 350 - 450 L/min (6 - 8 L/s)
↓ **PEF:** obstruction, restriction or older |
| MVV | **Maximum voluntary ventilation:** Patient breathes as hard and as fast as possible for 10, 12 or 15 s. Volume is noted and is multiplied by 6, 5 or 4 to extrapolate to 1 min. Up to 30% deviation is allowed | **Normal:**
120 - 180 L/min
↓ **MVV:**
obstruction & restriction
Estimated MVV = 35 x FEV1 |

NOTE: *Normal values referenced are for a young healthy person, aged 20 to 30 years.*

6.2.3   Flow-volume (F-V) loop

- FVC is displayed as a flow - volume spirogram, often referred to as flow - volume loop. Forced expiratory vital capacity (FEVC) is followed by forced inspiratory vital capacity (FIVC)
- F-V loops are useful because certain disorders produce characteristic shapes
- The vol versus t **curve** is an alternative way of presenting spirometric results

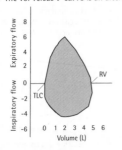

Fig. 13 Normal F-V loop

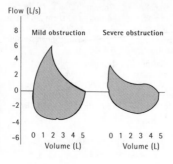

• Mild obstructive F-V loop is often caused by asthma/moderate COPD

• Severe obstructive F-V loop is characterized by decreased flows with very concaved inspiratory loop and increased expiration. Typical of emphysema

Fig. 14 Obstructive lung disease

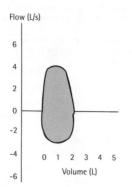

• Restrictive F-V loop is of normal shape, but of reduced size due to decreased lung volumes

• Restrictive lung disease is characterized by ↓ FEV_1 and FVC and normal or ↑ FEV_1/FVC ratio

Fig. 15 Restrictive lung disease

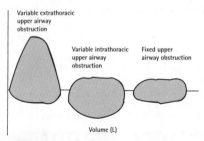

Fig. 16 Upper airway obstruction

1. **Variable extrathoracic upper airway obstruction** is characterized by normal expiratory flows and decreased inspiratory flows. It may be caused by vocal cord paralysis, thyromegaly or tracheamalacia

2. **Variable intrathoracic upper airway obstruction** is characterized by decreased expiratory flows and normal inspiratory flows. It may be caused by tracheal or bronchial tumor or tracheomalacia

3. **Fixed upper airway obstruction** is characterized by equal decrease in both inspiratory and expiratory flows, resulting in rectangular looking F-V loop. It may be due to tracheal stenosis, foreign body or vocal cord paralysis

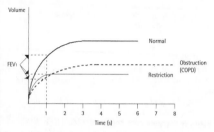

Fig. 17 Comparison of normal, obstructive and restrictive volume versus time curves

6.2.4   Other tests obtained using spirometry

Pre- and Post-bronchodilator spirometry

- After obtaining baseline spirometry, β_2 agonist is given via nebulizer and after 15 - 30 min spirometry is repeated
- ↑ FVC and/or FEV_1 by ≥ 12 - 15% and ≥ 200 ml = reversibility of airflow obstruction - consistent with asthma

Bronchial provocation

- After obtaining baseline spirometry, patient inhales bronchoconstricting agent such as methacholine and spirometry is repeated.
- ↓ FEV_1 by ≥ 20% below baseline = positive test for airway hyperreactivity

AARC Clinical Practice Guideline: Methacholine challenge testing

Description/definition:
- Patient inhales aerosol of methacholine
- Positive test = ↓ FEV_1 by 20% from baseline

Indications:
- Need to exclude diagnosis of airway hyperreactivity (e.g. asthma) to determine risk of developing asthma

Contraindications:
- *Absolute:*
  - FEV_1 < 50% of predicted or < 1 L
  - MI or CVA in last 3 months
  - Aortic or cerebral aneurysm
- Uncontrolled hypertension: American Thoracic Society (ATS) suggests sysBP > 200 mmHg and/or diaBP > 100 mmHg
- *Relative:*
  - FEV_1 > 50% or > 1.5 L but < 60% pred
  - Unable to perform acceptable spirometry
  - Upper or lower respiratory tract infection within previous 2-6 weeks
  - Current use of cholinesterase inhibitor medication (e.g. for myasthenia gravis)
  - Pregnancy and lactation
  - Failure to withhold medication may affect the test: recommended periods for withholding medication are generally based on duration of action
  - Foods that contain caffeine (coffee, tea, cola, chocolate) should be withheld on test day

Agent withholding time	
Short-acting β_2 agonist	6 - 8 h
Long-acting β_2 agonist (e.g. salmeterol, formoterol)	48 h
Anticholinergics: ipratropium (Atrovent), tiotropium	24 h up to 1 week
Disodium cromoglycate	8 h
Nedocromil	48 h
Oral β_2 agonists	24 h
Theophyllines	12 - 48 h
Leukotriene modifiers	24 h
Corticosteroids (inhaled or oral)	Unkown, may prolong

Hazards/Complications:
- Bronchoconstriction, hyperinflation, severe coughing
- Dizziness, light-headedness, chest pain
- Possible exposure of testing personnel to provocative substance

Resources:
- Equipment:
  - Spirometers must meet ATS requirements
  - Nebulizers used should produce aerosol 1 - 4 µm in size
  - Gas powering nebulizer must be set at correct pressure or flow (as per manufacturer's recommendations)
- Dosing: range 0.02 - 25 mg/ml diluted in sterile normal saline 0.9%
- Room with ≥ 2 complete air exchanges/h should be used to administer the test
- O_2, bronchodilators and resuscitation equipment must be readily available
- Personnel:
  - Physician trained in PFTs and experienced in bronchial provocation should direct testing
  - Recommended personnel performing these tests should hold Registered Respiratory Therapist (RRT)/Registered Pulmonary Function Technologists (RPFT) credentials (in the USA)

Patient monitoring:
- FEV_1 is the primary variable monitored
- Breath sounds, HR, pulse-ox, ± BP
- When > 20% fall in FEV_1, β_2 agonist may be given to speed up recovery

Frequency:
- 230 min should elapse before test repeated
- Tolerance to methacholine may occur in patients who are not asthmatic when test is repeated at < 24 h interval

American Association of Respiratory Care. Clinical Practice Guideline: Methacholine Challenge Testing: 2001 revision and update. Respir Care 2001; 46/5, 523 - 530.

6.3   Diffusion Capacity ($D_L CO$)

$D_L CO$ (also called **transfer factor**) is a test of A-C membrane effectiveness.

6.3.1   Technique

- Patient exhales to RV then inspires a gas mixture containing 0.3% carbon monoxide, 10% He, 21% O_2 and the remainder N_2 up to TLC, then holds their breath for 10 s
- Initial 1L of exhaled air is discarded and a sample of alveolar gas is taken and analyzed for CO and He

Normal value: 25 ml/min/mmHg; results within ± 20% of predicted are considered normal

6.3.2   Indications

- Evaluation and follow-up of parenchymal lung diseases: e.g. idiopathic pulmonary fibrosis (IPF), bronchiolitis obliterans organizing pneumonia (BOOP), diseases associated with dust, such as asbestosis
- Evaluation and follow-up of emphysema and cystic fibrosis and differentiating chronic bronchitis, emphysema and asthma in patients with obstructive patterns
- Quantification of importance and disability
- Evaluation of cardiovascular disease: primary pulmonary hypertension, acute or recurrent thromboembolism, pulmonary edema
- Evaluation of pulmonary involvement in systemic disease (e.g. systemic lupus erythematosus (SLE), rheumatoid arthritis)
- Evaluation of the effects of chemotherapy drugs or other drugs (e.g. amiodarone, bleomycin) known to induce pulmonary dysfunction
- Evaluation of pulmonary hemorrhage
- As an early indication of certain pulmonary infections (e.g. pneumocystis pneumonia)
- Prediction of arterial desaturation during exercise in some patients with lung disease

6.3.3   Contraindications

- **Absolute**
  - Carbon monoxide toxicity
  - Dangerous levels of oxyhemoglobin desaturation without supplemental O_2

- **Relative**
  - Mental confusion or muscular incoordination or inability to obtain/maintain adequate lip seal on the instrument mouthpiece
  - Large meal or vigorous exercise immediately before the test
  - Smoking within 24 h
  - ↓ Lung volumes that would not yield valid test results
  - Improperly calibrated or maintained devices

6.3.4   Assessment of test quality

- Test maneuvers and results should be evaluated according to ATS recommendations, in particular:
- Inspiratory volume > 90% of largest previously measured vital capacity (FVC or V$_C$), attained in < 2.5 s in healthy subjects and within 4 s in patients with mod-to-severe airway obstruction
- Breath-hold time 9 - 11 s, with no leaks or Valsava or Müller maneuvers
- Washout volume (dead space) should be 0.75 - 1L (or 0.5 if VC < 2 L)
- Volume of alveolar gas sample should be 0.5 - 1L obtained in < 4 s
- ≥ 2 acceptable tests should be averaged: D$_L$CO values should be reproducible to within 10% or 3 ml carbon monoxide/min/mmHg, whichever is greater
- Subject should have refrained from smoking for 24 h prior to test

NOTE: ≥ 4 min interval should elapse between maneuvers to allow test gas to be eliminated from lungs.

6.3.5   Factors that affect D$_L$CO results

Decreased D$_L$CO

- Loss of functioning A-C membrane with ↑ lung volume: emphysema
- Loss of functioning A-C membrane with ↓ lung volume:
  - Parenchymal restrictive processes (e.g. IPF, asbestosis, sarcoidosis, pneumonia)
  - Lung resection
- ↑COHb (smokers): this effect is ↓ by having patient not smoke for 24 h before test
- Pregnancy (1st trimester)
- Pulmonary circulation diseases (e.g. primary pulmonary hypertension, SLE)
- Anemia (↓ RBC)

Increased D_LCO

- ↑ Pulmonary blood flow (↑ RBC): exercise, pulmonary hemorrhage, L – R intracardiac shunt
- Polycythemia (e.g. COPD, CHF)

American Association of Respiratory Care. Clinical Practice Guideline: Single-breath Carbon Monoxide Diffusing Capacity. Respir Care 1999; 44: 539-546.

6.4 Summarizing Pulmonary Function Tests

	Measurement		
	normal	obstructive	restrictive
Lung volumes and capacities			
VT	500 – 600 ml	↑/N	↓/N
ERV	1 – 1.2 L	↓	↓
RV	1.2 – 1.5 L	↓	↓
IRV	2.5 – 3 L	↓	↓
TLC	5.5 – 6.5 L	↑	↓
IC	3 – 3.6 L	↓	↓
VC	4 – 5 L	↓	↓
FRC	2 – 2.5 L	↑	↓
Mechanics			
FVC	≥ 4 L	↓	↓
FEV_1	80% of FVC	↓	↓
FEV_3	97% of FVC	↓	↓
FEV_1/FVC	80%	↓	N/↑
$FEF_{25-75\%}$	4 – 6 L/s	↓	N/↓
PEF	500 – 600 L/min	↓	N/↓
MVV	120 – 180 L/min	↓	↓
Compliance	C_{stat} > 60 ml/cmH$_2$O	N/↑	↓

Resistance (R_{aw})	0.5 - 2.5 cmH$_2$O/ L/s	↑	N
MIP	70 - 100 cmH$_2$O	↓	↓
MEP	140 - 200 cmH$_2$O	↓	↓
Diffusion Capacity			
D$_L$CO	25 ml/min/mmHg	N (↓ in emphysema)	N/↓

BIBLIOGRAPHY

Crapo RO: Pulmonary Function Testing. In, Crapo JD et al (eds): Baum's Textbook of Pulmonary Diseases, 7th ed. LWW, 2004.

Grippi MA et al: Pulmonary Function Testing. In, Fishman AP et al (eds): Fishman's Pulmonary Diseases and Disorders, 3rd ed. McGraw-Hill 1997.

AARC Clinical Practice Guideline, Methacholine Challenge Testing: 2001 revision and update, Respir Care 2001; 46: 523-530.

7.   Cardiopulmonary Exercise Testing

7.1   Simple Tests of Exercise Capacity

7.1.1   Six-minute walk test (6 MWT)

- The subject walks as far as they can at their own pace for 6 min on a 30 m course (e.g. hospital corridor). He or she is free to stop and rest at any time. HR and SpO_2 are measured at baseline and at break intervals and recovery period
- This test evaluates global and integrated responses of all the systems involved during exercise. 6 MWT does not determine VO_2 peak, diagnose the cause of dyspnea on exertion or evaluate the causes of exercise limitation. Information provided by this test should complement cardiopulmonary exercise testing (CPET), not replace it
- Interpretation:
  - ↓ SpO_2 by > 5% indicates respiratory problem
  - ↑↑ HR without ↓ SpO_2 suggests unconditioned patient or cardiac problem

Indications
A. Pre- and Posttreatment comparison
Lung transplantation, lung resection, lung volume reduction surgery (LVRS), pulmonary rehabilitation, pulmonary hypertension, COPD and heart failure
B. Functional status
COPD, cystic fibrosis, heart failure, peripheral vascular disease, fibromyalgia and older patients
C. Morbidity and mortality predictor
Heart failure, COPD, primary pulmonary hypertension (PPH)

Contraindications
A. Absolute
Unstable angina during previous month and MI during previous month
B. Relative
Resting HR > 120/min; systolic BP > 180 mmHg; and diastolic BP > 100 mmHg

Safety issues

- Test should be performed where a rapid response is possible in case of emergency
- Supplies that must be available: O_2, sublingual nitroglycerine, aspirin and albuterol
- Must have telephone or other means of communication to enable patient to call for help
- Reasons for immediately stopping 6MWT: (1) chest pain; (2) intolerable dyspnea; (3) leg cramps; (4) staggering; (5) diaphoresis; and (6) pale or ashen appearance

American Thoracic Society Statement: Guidelines for the Six-minute Walk Test. Am J Respir Crit Care Med 2002; 166: 111-117.

7.1.2   Shuttle Test

- Measures the distance walked by an individual (back and forth from 2 points set 10 m apart) while being paced by audio cassette tape and the speed is progressively ↑
- Patient shuttles until cannot keep up with the tape or has to stop to recover his or her breath or for other reasons, such as with 6 MWT

7.1.3   Exercise testing for evaluation of hypoxemia and/or desaturation

Description/Definition

To determine the degree of O_2 desaturation and/or hypoxemia that occurs on exertion. Desaturation is defined as ↓ SaO_2 of 2%, $SaO_2 < 88\%$ and/or $PaO_2 \leq 55$ mmHg.

Indications

- To assess/quantify arterial HbO_2 saturation during exercise in patients suspected of desaturation (e.g. dyspnea on exertion, ↓ D_LCO, ↓ PaO_2 at rest or documented pulmonary disease)
- To quantify the response to therapeutic intervention (e.g. O_2 prescription, medications, smoking cessation) or to reassess the need for continued supplemental O_2 therapy
- To titrate optimal amount of O_2 therapy for hypoxemia or desaturation during activity

- Preoperative assessment for lung resection or transplant
- To assess degree of impairment for disability evaluation (e.g. asbestosis, pneumoconiosis)

Contraindications

A. Absolute	B. Relative
• Acute serious EKG changes	• When pulse oximetry may provide invalid data (e.g. ↑ HbCO, HbMet or ↓ perfusion)
• Uncontrolled CHF, asthma or systemic hypertension	
• MI within previous 4 weeks	• Arterial puncture ± arterial cannulation may be contraindicated
• Recent or acute thromboembolism or DVT	• Patient unable or unwilling to perform test
• Pulmonary edema	• Severe PH/cor pulmonale
• Respiratory failure	• Resting sysBP > 200 mmHg or diaBP > 100 mmHg
• 2° or 3° heart block	• SaO_2 < 85% on room air
• Symptomatic severe aortic stenosis	• Neuromuscular, musculoskeletal or rheumatoid disorders exacerbated by exercise
• Aneurysm of heart or aorta	
• Unstable angina, acute pericarditis or myocarditis	• Uncontrolled metabolic disease (e.g. diabetes)
• Acute non-cardiopulmonary disorders affected by exercise	• Complicated or advanced pregnancy
	• Unable to cooperate/follow directions

Precautions and/or possible complications

- Indications for immediate termination:
  - EKG abnormalities (e.g. dangerous dysrhythmias, V-tach, ST-T wave changes)
  - Severe desaturation: $SaO_2 \leq 80\%$ or $SpO_2 \leq 83\%$ and/or 10% fall from baseline
  - Angina
  - Hypotensive response (↓ sysBP > 20 mmHg occurring after normal exercise rise) or (↓ sysBP < pre-exercise level)
  - Lightheadedness
  - Request from patient to end the test

- Abnormal responses that may require discontinuation of exercise include:
  (1) sysBP > 250 mmHg or diaBP > 120 mmHg or ↑ sysBP < 20 mmHg from resting level
  (2) mental confusion or headache
  (3) cyanosis
  (4) nausea or vomiting
  (5) muscle cramping

Limitations of procedure/validation of results

- Limitations of pulse oximetry:
  - Overestimation of SpO_2 with HbCO > 4%
  - ↓ SpO_2 accuracy with desaturations < 83%
  - ↓ perfusion may ⇒ false +ve results or no valid data; evaluate for alternative site (e.g. ear, forehead)
  - Motion artifact ⇒ no readout
  - Underestimation of SpO_2 may result when Hb ≤ 8 g/dl
- Validation of results:
  - ABG samples should be obtained at rest and at peak exercise
  - Validity of pulse oximetry is verified by comparison of CO-oximetry results

American Association of Respiratory Care Guideline: Exercise Testing for Evaluation of Hypoxemia and/or Desaturation. Respir Care 2001; 46: 514-522.

7.2   Progressive Exercise Testing

Cardiopulmonary exercise testing (CPET) provides a global assessment of the integrative exercise response of pulmonary, cardiovascular, NM and other systems that is not adequately reflected through the measurement of individual organ system function.

Indications

a. Evaluation of exercise intolerance

Determination of functional impairment/capacity (VO_2peak) and/or exercise-limiting factors

b. Evaluation of undiagnosed exercise intolerance

- Unexplained dyspnea when initial test results are nondiagnostic
- Assessing contribution of cardiopulmonary cause in coexisting etiology

c. Evaluation of patients with cardiovascular disease

Assessment of exercise capacity and response to therapy of patients with heart failure who are being considered for heart transplantation

d. Evaluation of patients with respiratory disease

- COPD: establishing exercise limitations and magnitude of hypoxemia and for oxygen prescription
- Interstitial lung disease: detection of early gas exchange abnormalities and magnitude of hypoxemia for O_2 prescription and documenting therapeutic response to potential toxic therapy
- Pulmonary vascular disease, cystic fibrosis and exercise-induced bronchospasm

e. Other applications

- Preoperative evaluation (lung resection, ± LVRS for emphysema)
- Evaluation for impairment/disability
- Evaluation for prescription for pulmonary rehabilitation
- Evaluation for lung or heart-lung transplantation

Contraindications

a. Absolute

- Acute MI (3 - 5 days)
- Uncontrolled symptomatic arrhythmias, CHF and/or asthma
- $SpO_2 \leq 85\%$ on room air
- Mental impairment $\Rightarrow$ unable to cooperate
- Endocarditis, myocarditis or pericarditis
- Severe symptomatic aortic stenosis
- Respiratory failure
- Acute pulmonary embolism/DVT or pulmonary infarction
- Acute noncardiopulmonary disorder that may affect CPET performance or be aggravated by CPET
- Syncope

b. Relative

- Severe systematic hypertension: sysBP > 200 mmHg, diaBP > 120 mmHg
- Significant pulmonary hypertension
- Hypertrophic cardiomyopathy
- Tachy-or bradyarrhythmias
- High degree AV block
- Advanced/complicated pregnancy
- Electrolyte abnormalities
- Orthopedic impairment
- Stenotic valvular heart disease or coronary stenosis

Criteria For Exercise Termination

- $SpO_2 \leq 80\%$ with signs and symptoms of severe hypoxemia
- Loss of coordination, sudden pallor, mental confusion, dizziness or faintness
- Hypertension: sysBP > 250 mmHg; diaBP > 120 mmHg
- ↓ sysBP > 20 mmHg from highest value during test
- Chest pain
- Signs of respiratory failure
- 2° or 3° heart block or ischemic EKG changes

Modes of exercise

a. Treadmill

- Motor-driven; imposes progressively ↑ exercise stress through a combination of speed and grade increases
- More appropriate for athletes; on average, maximum oxygen consumption (VO_2max) is ~ 5 - 10% higher than on cycle ergometer

b. Cycle ergometer

- Less expensive and requires less space than treadmill. Main advantage over treadmill: external work rate is measurable
- Appropriate for patients. In most clinical situations, it is preferable over treadmill

Measurements

a. Oxygen uptake (VO_2)

- **VO_2max:** best index of aerobic capacity and the gold standard of cardiopulmonary fitness. It represents oxygen consumption at maximum exertion
- **VO_2peak:** often used as an estimate of VO_2max
- **Normal VO_2max:** is > 84%. Treadmill values are ~ 10% > cycle ergometry values
- **Increased VO_2max:** VO_2 can increase from its resting normal value of ~ 3.5 ml/kg (~ 250 ml/min) to VO_2max of ~ 30 - 50 ml/min/kg (~ 15 x normal value) Athletes: > 80 ml/min/kg (20 x resting value)
- **Decreased VO_2max:** reflects O_2 transport problems (e.g. CO, O_2-carrying capacity of blood, pulmonary and/or NM limitations) and effort. Indicates decreased exercise capacity

b. Carbon dioxide output (VCO_2)

- Determined by factors similar to those of VO_2. During progressive exercise, VCO_2 (carbon dioxide production) increases nearly as much as VO_2

c. Respiratory exchange ratio (RER)

- RER = VCO_2/VO_2 ratio. Measured by gas exchange at mouth; used as a rough estimate of metabolic events (RQ). Under steady conditions, RER ≈ RQ
- Meaning of RER (RQ) values: ~ 1: mainly metabolism of carbohydrates 0.8: protein metabolism 0.7: fat metabolism> 1: consider either lactic acidosis or hyperventilation

d. Anaerobic threshold (AT)

- AT estimates the onset of metabolic acidosis associated with increased arterial lactate during exercise. AT is helpful as an indicator of level of fitness, for exercise prescription and to monitor effect of physical training
- Normal value: occurs at ~ 50 - 70% of VO_2 (wide range of normal: 35 - 80%)
- Decreased AT: can be due to many nonspecific conditions; need to examine other measurements to determine underlying etiology
- AT < 40% of predicted VO_2max may indicate pulmonary (desaturation) or other limitations in O_2 supply to tissues or mitochondrial abnormality

e. Cardiac output (CO)

- CO is not routinely measured
- Can be calculated by Fick equation: $CO = VO_2/C(a - v)O_2$

f. Heart rate (HR)

- HR normally increases linearly with increases in VO_2
- HR_{max} equation for predicted HR: 220 - age or 210 - (age x 0.65)
- HR_{peak}: decreased in many patients with cardiopulmonary diseases
- $HR_{reserve}$ (HRR): = predicted HR - HR; should be < 15 beats/min and HR% of predicted should be > 90

g. Oxygen pulse (VO_2/HR ratio)

- Reflects the amount of O_2 extracted/HR. May estimate stroke volume (SV) during exercise. **Normal** O_2 pulse: > 80%
- **Increased:** incremental exercise due to increased SV and O_2 extraction
  Decreased: deconditioning or early exercise limitation due to ventilatory constraint

h. Blood pressure (BP)

- If BP does not increase with exercise or it decreases, a cardiac limitation or abnormality of sympathetic control is suggested
- If BP decreases as exercise intensity increases, the test should be terminated immediately. Marked increase in BP is often seen in patients with resting hypertension

i. Ventilatory reserve (VR)

- Corresponds to how close peak V_E (ventilatory demand) achieved during exercise ($V_E$max) approaches MVV (ventilatory capacity) or some estimate of MVV (FEV_1 x 35 or 40). Normal: < 85%
- Decreased VR: pulmonary disease (decreased MVV, increased V_E)

Other variables measured during CPET include:
- Maximum expiratory pressures (MEP)
- Minimum expiratory pressures (MIP), V_D/V_T, $P(A - a)O_2$

ATS/ACCP Statement on Cardiopulmonary Exercise Testing. Am J Respir Crit Care Med 2003; 167: 211–277.

7.2.1   Basic response patterns in exercise testing

Variable	Abbr.	Respiratory disease	Cardiac disease	Deconditioned
Maximal O_2 uptake	VO_2max	↓	↓	↓
Heart rate, peak	HR_{peak}	↓	Variable	Norm/↓
Anaerobic threshold	AT	Norm/↓	↓	Norm/↓
Oxygen pulse	O_2pulse	Norm/↓	↓	↓
Ventilatory reserve (V_E/MVV) x 100	VR	Norm/↑	Norm/↓	Normal
Wasted ventilation	V_D/V_T	↑	↑	Normal
Arterial O_2 tension	PaO_2	Variable	Normal	Normal
Alveolar to arterial O_2 tension difference	$P(A-a)O_2$	↑	Normal	Normal

RESPIRATORY DISEASES

8.   Obstructive Lung Diseases

8.1   Asthma

Definition
- Asthma is a chronic inflammatory disease of the airways resulting in airflow obstruction secondary to airway edema, increased mucus production, bronchospasm and infiltration of the airway with leukocytes (eosinophils, lymphocytes and neutrophils). It is usually reversible either spontaneously or with treatment
- **Status asthmaticus:** severe acute asthma attack refractory to optimal treatment which may require ventilatory support

Statistics
- **Prevalence:** affects ~ 5% of US population (up to 10% of children) and ≥ 10% of the world population
- **Mortality:** 5000 - 6000 deaths/year

Etiology
- **Allergic:** begins early in life; results from exposure to antigens such as pollen, certain foods, smoke, pollutants ⇒ IgE activation ⇒ antigen- antibody reaction involving pulmonary inflammatory response; genetic
- **Nonallergic:** usually of later onset (> 35 years); secondary to respiratory infections, anxiety, irritant gases, pollutants, exercise in cold weather, large changes in Pb and temperature, strong emotion (laughing, crying, etc) and drugs (aspirin, β-blockers)

Pathology
- Many cells (mastcells, lymphocytes, macrophages, etc.) and their mediators (histamine, leukotrienes, etc) play a role in causing bronchoconstriction and edema, resulting in ↓ airway diameter and ↑ R_{aw}
- Pathological changes:
  (1) Hypertrophy of airway smooth muscle
  (2) Hyperplasia of mucus glands and goblet cells ⇒ hypersecretion
  (3) Inflammation (edema)
  (4) Subepithelial collagen deposition (airway remodeling) in some patients
      = airflow obstruction; may be partially reversible

Clinical manifestations

Signs and symptoms:
- **Dyspnea**
- **Wheezing** (all that wheezes is NOT asthma; wheezing may also occur with COPD, CHF, aspiration, upper airway obstruction and vocal cord dysfunction)
- **Cough**
- **Chest tightness**
- Tachypnea
- Tachycardia
- Restlessness
- Accessory muscle use
- Retractions in children
- ± Cyanosis, diaphoresis
- ↑ **Expiratory time**
- Pulsus paradoxus: ↓ sysBP by > 10 mmHg on inspiration

ABG:
↓ PaO_2, ↓ $PaCO_2$ (↑ in severe attack)

PFT:
- ↓ **Expiratory flows:** ↓ FVC, FEV_1, FEV_1/FVC
- ↑ **Lung volumes:** ↑ RV, TLC, FRC, secondary to air trapping
- **Normal D_LCO**

Diagnosis

- **Bronchoprovocation test:** test for airway hyperreactivity. Patient inhales progressively higher doses of bronchoconstricting agent such as histamine or methacholine. After each dose, FEV_1 is measured and dose that causes ↓ FEV_1 by 20% is known as provocative dose (PD 20). → p. 64
- **Pre- and post-bronchodilator:** ↑ FEV_1 by > 12 - 15% and > 200 ml = reversible obstruction
- **D_LCO:** normal in asthma (and chronic bronchitis); ↓ in emphysema

Monitoring

- **Peak expiratory flow rate (PEFR):**
  - Difference of > 20% between morning and afternoon PEFR may suggest asthma (note: normal PEFR ≥ 400 - 600 L/min)
  - **Severe bronchospasm:** PEFR < 100 L/min
  - **Extreme danger:** PEFR < 60 L/min

- **Sputum eosinophilia:** marker of airway inflammation; asthmatic patients with higher sputum eosinophilia are likely to benfit from corticosteroid therapy
- **Exhaled nitric oxide:** higher exhaled nitric oxide levels predict airway inflammation and poor asthmatic control

Differential diagnosis

- **COPD:** may coexist with asthma or it may have a reversible component
- **Pulmonary edema** (cardiac asthma)
- **Large airway obstruction:** foreign body, tumor, tracheal stenosis, vocal cord dysfunction
- May also consider: cystic fibrosis, bronchiolitis, pneumonias (aspiration), pulmonary emboli, laryngomalacia
- In children, it is distinguished from bronchiolitis because it responds to bronchodilators

Treatment

1. Prevent:
Attacks by avoiding triggers

2. Oxygen:
For hypoxemia

3. Quick relief medications:
- Short-acting β_2 agonists (albuterol, levalbuterol, metaproterenol) are 1st line defense for acute attack
- Anticholinergics (Atrovent) are 2nd line defense which may be added to β_2 agonist, possibly enhancing actions of the latter
- Systemic corticosteroids (prednisone, prednisolone, methylprednisolone) for acute exacerbations nonresponsive to bronchodilators
- $\pm$ Theophylline

4. Long-term control medications:
- **Inhaled corticosteroids** (beclovent, budesonide, fluticasone) to prevent long-term symptoms. Spacer should be used and mouth rinsed after dose to ↓ risk of oral candidiadis
- **Long-term β_2 agonist** (salmeterol [Serevent]) may be useful in nocturnal asthma
- **Theophylline** as an adjunct to anti-inflammatory drugs
- **Cromolyn sodium** may be useful for allergy and exercise-induced asthma

○ **Anti-leukotrienes** may be of use in mild asthma:
- Accolate (Zafirlukast)
- Singulair (Montelukast)
- Zyflo (Zileuton)

○ **Xolair (Omalizumab):**
Binds to circulating IgE antibodies ⇒ ↓ amount of IgE antibodies available to bind to mast cells. Therefore, it blocks allergic reactions
- Indication: patients > 12 years old with moderate-to-severe persistent (allergic) asthma who get very little or no relief from standard asthma medications
- Dose: 1-2 vials/month SC

5. Heliox:

A mixture of helium and oxygen (80% helium: 20% oxygen or 70% helium: 30% oxygen) is a controversial alternative therapy for severe acute asthma attack. It is usually administered in the emergency department. See chapter on medical gases for further information on He-O_2 gas therapy.

6. Intubation/MV:

○ For respiratory failure (RF) and status asthmaticus
○ Only about 5% of all hospitalized asthma patients require intubation and mechanical ventilation and most intubated patients usually recover rapidly with treatment; most of these patients can be extubated within 2 - 3 days
○ **Predictors:**
- Severe hypoxemia on $FIO_2 > 0.5$, $PaCO_2 > PaO_2$, pH < 7.25
- ↓/absent breath sounds
- PEFR < 50%
- Nasal flaring and RR > 40/min in children
○ **Goals of mechanical ventilation:**
Provide acceptable gas exchange and avoid air trapping. This pulmonary hyperinflation can lead to hypotension. Generally, V_T of 5 - 8 ml/kg (maintain $P_{plat} < 30$ cmH$_2$O) and inspiratory flow > 80 L/min help reduce the risk of alveolar overdistension and air trapping

7. Stepwise approach for managing asthma in adults and children > 5 years old

Classify severity: clinical feature before treatment or adequate control			Medications required to maintain long-term control
	Symptoms/day PEF or FEV$_1$ **Symptoms/night PEF** **variability**		**Daily medications** (dark gray shaded areas = preferred treatment)
STEP 4 severe persistent	Continual Frequent	≤ 60% > 30%	• High-dose inhaled corticosteroid AND • Long-acting inhaled β$_2$ agonist
			AND, if needed, • Corticosteroid tablets or syrup long term (2 mg/kg/d, not > 60 mg/d). [Make repeat attempts to ↓ systemic corticosteroids and maintain control with high-dose inhaled corticosteroids]
STEP 3 moderate persistent	Daily > 1 night/ week	> 60%-< 80% > 30%	• Low-to medium-dose inhaled corticosteroids AND long-acting inhaled β$_2$ agonists
			• ↑ inhaled corticosteroids within medium-dose range OR • Low-to medium-dose inhaled corticosteroids AND either leukotriene modifier or theophylline

STEP 3 moderate persistent	Daily > 1 night/ week	$\geq 60\% - < 80\%$ > 30%	If needed: recurring severe exacerbations • ↑ inhaled corticosteroids within medium-dose range AND add long-acting inhaled β_2 agonist OR alternatively • ↑ inhaled corticosteroids within medium-dose range AND add either leukotriene modifier or theophylline
STEP 2 mild persistent	≥ 2/week < 1/day ≥ 2 nights/month	$\geq 80\%$ 20-30%	• Low-dose inhaled corticosteroids • Cromolyn, leukotriene modifier, nedocromil or sustained release theophylline to serum concentration of 5 - 15 µg/ml
STEP 1 mild intermit-tent	≤ 2 days/week ≤ 2 nights/month	$\geq 80\%$ < 20%	• No daily medications needed • Severe exacerbations may occur, separated by long periods of normal lung function and no symptoms. A course of systemic corticosteroids is recommended

Quick relief: all patients:
- Short-acting inhaled β_2 agonist bronchodilator:
  2 - 4 puffs as needed for symptoms
- Intensity of treatment will depend on severity of exacerbation:
  up to 3 treatments at 20 min intervals or a single nebulizer treatment as needed. Course of systemic corticosteroids may also be needed
- Use of short-acting β_2 agonists > 2 x/week in intermittent asthma may indicate the need to initiate (increase) long-term therapy

NOTES:
- *Step down:* Review treatment every 1 - 6 months; a gradual stepwise reduction in treatment may be possible
- *Step up:* If control is not maintained, consider step up. First, review patient medications technique, adherence and environmental control
- The stepwise approach is meant to assist, not replace, the clinical decision-making required to meet individual patient needs
- Refer to asthma specialist if there are difficulties controlling asthma or if step 4 care is required

Source: NIH Expert Report Panel 2, Guidelines Publications (Selected Update of 1997 Guidelines) No. 97-4051 2002.

8. Stepwise approach for managing infants and young children < 5 years old with acute or chronic asthma

Classify severity: clinical features before treatment or adequate control		Medications required to maintain long-term control
	Symptoms/day **Symptoms/night**	**Daily medications** (dark gray shaded areas = preferred therapy)
STEP 4 **severe** **persistent**	<u>Continual</u> Frequent	• High-dose inhaled corticosteroids AND long-acting inhaled β_2 agonist
		AND, if needed, • Corticosteroid tablets or syrup long term (2 mg/kg/d, not > 60 mg/d). [Make repeat attempts to ↓ systemic corticosteroids and maintain control with high-dose inhaled corticosteroids]
STEP 3 **moderate** **persistent**	<u>Daily</u> > 1 night/week	• Low-dose inhaled corticosteroids and long-acting inhaled β_2 agonist OR • Medium-dose inhaled corticosteroids

STEP 3 moderate persistent	Daily > 1 night/week	• Low-dose inhaled corticosteroids AND either leukotriene receptor antagonist or theophylline If needed: recurring severe exacerbations • Medium-dose inhaled corticosteroid and long-acting β_2 agonist OR, alternatively, • Medium-dose inhaled corticosteroids and either leukotriene receptor antagonist or theophylline
STEP 2 mild persistent	≥ 2/week but < 1/day > 2 nights/month	• Low-dose inhaled corticosteroid (with nebulizer or metered-dose inhaler [MDI] with holding chamber with or without face mask or dry powder inhalers [DPI]) • Cromolyn (nebulizer preferred or MDI with holding chamber) OR leukotriene receptor anatagonist
STEP 1 mild intermittent	≤ 2 days/week ≤ 2 nights/month	• No daily medications needed

Quick relief: all patients
- Bronchodilator as needed for symptoms; preferred: **short-acting inhaled β_2 agonist** by nebulizer or face mask and space/holding chamber; alternative: **oral β_2 agonist**
- With viral respiratory infection: bronchodilator q4 - 6 h up to 24 h (longer with physician consult); generally, repeat no more than once every 6 weeks. Consider systemic corticosteroid if exacerbation is severe or patient has history of previous severe exacerbations
- Use of short-acting β_2 agonists > 2 x/week in intermitt. asthma (or ↑ use in persistent asthma) may indicate need to initiate (increase) long-term controlling therapy

NOTE: *Same as for stepwise approach in adults and children > 5 years old; also, there are very few studies on asthma therapy for infants.*

Source: NIH Expert Panel Report 2, Guidelines Publications (Selected Update of 1997 Guidelines) No. 97- 4051 2002.

9. Usual dosages for long-term control medications

Medication	Dosage form	Adult dose	Child dose*
Inhaled corticosteroids (See estimated daily dosages for inhaled corticosteroids below)			
Systemic corticosteroids	**(applies to all 3 corticosteroids)**		
Methyl-prednisolone	2, 4, 8, 16, 32 mg tab	7.5 - 60 mg/d	0.25 - 2 mg/kg/d
Prednisolone	5 mg tab 5 mg/5 ml 15 mg/5 ml	• Daily in single dose or qod. as needed for control • Short-course 'burst':	
Prednisone	1, 2.5, 10, 20, 50 mg tab; 5 mg/ml, 5 mg/5 ml	adult: 40 - 60 mg/d single dose or 2 divided doses for 3 - 10 days; child: 1 - 2 mg/kg/d max 60 mg/d for 3 - 10 days	
Long-acting inhaled β_2 agonists (Should not be used for symptom relief or exacerbations. Use with inhaled corticosteroids)			
Salmeterol	MDI 21 µg/puff DPI 50 µg/blister	2 puff q12 h 1 blister q12 h	1 - 2 puffs q12 h 1 blister q12 h
Formoterol	DPI 12 µg/single use capsule	1 capsule q12 h	1 capsule q12 h
Combined medications			
Fluticasone/ Salmeterol	DPI 100, 250 or 500 µg/50 µg	1 inhalation bid; dose depends on asthma severity	1 inhalation bid; dose depends on asthma severity
Cromolyn and Nedocromil			
Cromolyn	MDI 1 mg/puff Nebulizer 20 mg/ampule	2 - 4 puffs tid -qid 1 ampule tid - qid	1 - 2 puffs tid - qid 1 ampule tid - qid
Nedocromil	MDI 1.75 mg/ 50 µg	2 - 4 puffs bid - qid	1 - 2 puffs bid - qid

Leukotriene Modifiers

Montelukast	4 or 5 chewable tablets 10 mg tablet	10 mg qhs	4 mg qhs (2 - 5 years) 5 mg qhs (6 - 14 years) 10 mg qhs (> 14 years)
Zafirlukast	10 or 20 mg tab	40 mg/day (20 mg tab bid)	20 mg/day (7 - 11 years) (10 mg tablet bid)
Zileuton	300 or 600 mg tab	2400 mg/d (tablet qid)	

Methylxanthines
(target serum concentration of 5 - 15 µg/ml at steady state)

Theophylline	Liquids, sustained release tablets and capsules	Starting dose 10 mg/kg/d up to 300 mg max; usual max 800 mg/d	Starting dose 10 mg/kg/d; usual max: < 1 year: 0.2 (age in weeks) + 5 = mg/kg/d > 1 year: 16 mg/kg/d

*Children ≤ 12 years of age

10. Estimated comparative daily dosages for inhaled corticosteroids

Drug	Low daily dose Adult/Child*	Medium daily dose Adult/Child*	High daily dose Adult/Child*
Beclomethasone CFC 42 or 84 µg/puff	168 - 504 µg 84 - 336 µg	504 - 840 µg 336 - 672 µg	> 840 µg > 672 µg
Beclomethasone HFA 40 or 80 µg/puff	80 - 240 µg 80 - 160 µg	240 - 480 µg 160 - 320 µg	> 480 µg > 320 µg
Budesonide DPI 200 µg/inhalation Nebulizer solution (child)	200 - 600 µg 200 - 400 µg 0.5 µg	600 - 1,200 µg 400 - 800 µg 1 µg	> 1200 µg > 800 µg 2 µg

Flunisolide	500 – 1000 µg	1000 – 2000 µg	> 2000 µg
250 µg/puff	500 – 750 µg	1000 – 1250 µg	> 1250 µg
Fluticasone	88 – 264 µg	264 – 660 µg	> 660 µg
MDI: 44, 110,	88 – 176 µg	176 – 440 µg	> 440 µg
210 µg/puff			
DPI: 50,100,	100 – 300 µg	300 – 600 µg	> 600 µg
250 µg/inh	100 – 200 µg	200 – 400 µg	> 400 µg
Triamcinolone	400 – 1000 µg	1000 – 2000 µg	> 2000 µg
acetonide	400 – 800 µg	800 – 1200 µg	> 1200 µg
100 µg/puff			

*Children ≤ 12 years of age

11. Managing asthma exacerbations: emergency department and hospital-based care (NIH 1997)

History, physical examination (breath sounds [BS], accessory muscle use, HR, RR), O_2sat, PEF or FEV_1

↓ | ↓ | ↓

FEV_1 or PEF > 50%
- β_2 agonist by MDI or nebulizer up to 3 x in 1st hour
- O_2 to keep O_2sat ≥ 90%
- Oral steroids if no immediate response

FEV_1 or PEF < 50%
- High-dose β_2 agonist + anticholinergic by nebulizer q20 min or continuous x 1 h
- O_2 to keep O_2sat ≥ 90%
- Oral (PO) steroids

Impending respiratory arrest
- Intubation + MV with 100% O_2
- β_2 agonist + anticholinergic nebulizer
- IV steroids

↓ | ↓

Repeat examination, PEF, O_2sat, other tests as needed

Admit to ICU

↓ | ↓

Moderate exacerbation
- FEV_1 or PEF 50 - 80% of predicted/best
- Moderate symptoms
- Inhaled β_2 agonist q60 min
- Oral or ↑ inhaled steroids
- Treat 1 - 3h if improvement

Severe exacerbation
- FEV_1 or PEF < 50% of predict./best
- Severe symptoms at rest
- No improvement after initial treatment
- Inhaled β_2 agonist q1h or contin. + inh. anticholinergic
- O_2 and syst. steroids

↓ | ↓ | ↓

Good response	Incomplete response	Poor response
• FEV_1 or PEF ≥ 70% x 1 h • Normal exam; no distress	• FEV_1 or PEF ≥ 50% & < 70% • Mild-moderate symptoms	• FEV_1 or PEF < 50% • PCO_2 ≥ 42 mmHg • Severe symptoms
↓	OR ↓ (individualize)	↓
Discharge home • Continue inhaled β_2 agonist + oral steroid course • Patient education: review medications, plan, follow-up	Admit to hospital ward • Inhaled β_2 agonist and anticholinergic • Systemic steroids (PO or IV) • O_2 • Monitor FEV_1 or PEF, HR, O_2sat	Admit to ICU • Inhaled β_2 agonist q1 h or cont. + inhaled anticholinergic • IV steroids • O_2 • Possible intubation + MV

8.2   Chronic Obstructive Pulmonary Disease (COPD)

Progressive airflow obstruction (↓ expiratory flow) which may be partially reversible, unlike the reversible airway obstruction found in asthma.

Includes chronic bronchitis or emphysema or both and sometimes asthma that has an irreversible component.

8.2.1   Chronic bronchitis

- **Defined clinically** as a chronic productive cough on most days for ≥ 3 months for ≥ 2 consecutive years
- It causes airflow limitation by narrowing the airways with mucosal thickening and excessive amounts of mucus due to hyperplasia of mucus producing glands

8.2.2   Emphysema

- **Defined histologically** as the permanent dilation of air spaces distal to terminal bronchioles by destruction of alveolar walls/lung parenchyma ⇒ ↓ elasticity
- It causes airway obstruction by ↓ elasticity (elastic recoil) = airways close prematurely on expiration. Normally, elastic recoil holds the airways inflated on expiration
- Patients who have pure emphysema uncomplicated by chronic bronchitis have irreversible airflow obstruction

Statistics

- 4th leading cause of death in the USA and the world
- $\geq$ 15 million people have COPD in USA, of whom about 2 million have emphysema; however, most people with COPD have features of both chronic bronchitis and emphysema

Etiology

- **Cigarette smoking** accounts for ~ 90% of COPD cases, but only ~ 15% of smokers develop COPD. This indicates that host factors play a role in the pathophysiology of the disease (Genetics? Varied patient resistance to infections?)
- Pollutants, prolonged exposure to chemicals and chronic recurrent respiratory infections also play a role
- **Genetics:** hereditary α-1 antitrypsin deficiency is a rare cause and is found in ~ 1% of emphysema patients. This figure may be higher because many patients with α-1 antitrypsin deficiency go undiagnosed and are treated simply as patients with emphysema. α-1 Antitrypsin is an enzyme that metabolizes trypsin, a digestive enzyme, which if not metabolized causes destruction of lung tissue

NOTE: Not all patients with α-1 antitrypsin deficiency develop emphysema, especially if they are not exposed to cigarettes.

Pathophysiology

- $\uparrow$ No. of mucus glands and goblet cells and $\uparrow$ size of mucus glands
  = hypersecretion $\Rightarrow$ airway obstruction
- Ciliary impairment as a result of exposure to smoke and infections
  $\Rightarrow$ $\downarrow$ mucociliary clearance $\Rightarrow$ medium for infections and airway plugs
- Inflammation (mucosal edema) and chronic cough
- **Emphysema:** inflammation and irritation (smoking) recruits inflammatory cells which produce elastase that destroys connective tissue around alveoli
  $\Rightarrow$ $\downarrow$ elastic recoil that drives air out
- Airway obstruction from hypersecretion and inflammation
  $\Rightarrow$ $\uparrow$ V/Q mismatch and hypoxemia

Clinical manifestations

Feature	Chronic bronchitis 'Blue Bloater'	Emphysema 'Pink Puffer'
	Fig. 18 Blue Bloater	Fig. 19 Pink Puffer
Age at diagnosis	> 50 years	> 60 years
Smoking	Common	Common
Cough	Chronic, productive	Little
Dyspnea	Mild, variable	Severe, progressive
Sputum	Large, purulent	Little
Infections	Frequent, recurrent	Less often
Chest	Normal, accessory muscle use	↑ A-P diameter secondary to hyperinflation; hypertrophied accessory muscles
Body	Stocky or fat	Thin
Breath sounds	Rhonchi, wheezing	↓, ↑ expiratory time (Te) ± wheezing
CXR	↑ Vascular markings; cardiomegaly	Hyperinflation, flat diaphragm and small heart silhouette
ABG PaO_2 $PaCO_2$ pH	45 - 60 mmHg (marked ↓) 50 - 60 mmHg (chronic ↑) compensated resp. acidosis	60 - 75 mmHg (mild ↓) 30 - 40 mmHg (normal or ↓) normal or ↑
Cyanosis	Yes: blue	Rare: pink

Cor pulmonale	Common	Rare
Hematocrit	> 50 - 55 (polycythemia)	35 - 45
PFT Lung volume Expir. flows Compliance $D_L CO$	↑ TLC, FRC, RV ↓ FVC, FEV_1, FEV_1/FVC Normal Normal	↑ FRC, RV, TLC ↓ FVC, FEV_1, FEV_1/FVC ↑ ↓ secondary to loss of A-C membrane
pH	More often	Less often

NOTE: *Many patients have features of both conditions; better long-term survival in patients with hypercapnia (blue bloater), paradoxically.*

8.3 Components of COPD Management [GOLD guidelines]

8.3.1 Component 1: Assess and monitor Disease

Diagnosis

Consider diagnosis of COPD in any patient who has chronic cough, chronic sputum production or dyspnea that is progressive, persistent or worse on exercise and/or history of exposure to risk factors for the disease (e.g. tobacco smoke, occupational dust and chemicals and/or smoke from cooking/heating fuels).
The diagnosis is confirmed by spirometry.

- **Physical examination:** rarely diagnostic in COPD. Physical signs of airflow limitation are usually absent until significant impairment of lung function has occurred
- **Spirometry:**
  - In order to identify patients earlier in the course of COPD, spirometry should be performed for patients with chronic cough and sputum production and history of exposure to risk factors (even if not dyspneic)
  - COPD patients typically have ↓ in both FEV_1 and FVC
  - **Postbronchodilator FEV_1** < 80% of predicted and FEV_1/FVC < 70% confirms airflow limitation that is not fully reversible

- The following investigations may be useful for patients in Stage II
  - moderate COPD:
    - **Bronchodilator reversibility test:** useful to rule out asthma
    - **Glucocorticosteroid reversibility testing:** a trial of 6 weeks to 3 months of inhaled glucocorticosteroids is used, in order to identify patients likely to respond to long-term glucocorticosteroids. FEV_1 ↑ of ≥ 200 ml and 12% = glucocorticosteroid reversibility
- **Chest X-ray:** seldom diagnostic unless obvious bullous disease is present
- **ABG:** should be done in patients with FEV_1 < 40% predicted or with clinical signs suggestive of respiratory failure or right heart failure
- **Alpha-1 antitrypsin deficiency screening:** may be of value in COPD patients < 45 year old or those that have family history of the disease
- **Differential diagnosis:** see table below

Diagnosis	Suggestive features (not in every case)
COPD	• Onset in midlife • Slowly progressive symptoms • Dyspnea during exercise • Largely irreversible airflow limitation
Asthma	• Onset early in life (often childhood) • Symptoms vary from day to day • Symptoms at night/early morning • Allergy, rhinitis and/or eczema also present • Family history • Largely reversible airflow limitation
Congestive heart failure (CHF)	• Fine basilar crackles • CXR shows dilated heart, pulmonary edema • PFTs indicate restriction, not airflow limitation
Bronchiectasis	• Large volumes of purulent sputum • Commonly associated with bacterial infection • Coarse crackles • Clubbing • CXR/CT show bronchial dilation, bronchial wall thickening

Tuberculosis	• Onset at all ages • CXR shows lung infiltrate or nodular lesions • Microbiological confirmation • High local prevalence for TB
Obliterative Bronchiolitis	• Onset in younger age, nonsmokers • Possibly history of rheumatoid arthritis • CT on expiration shows hypodense areas
Diffuse Panbronchiolitis	• Mostly male and nonsmokers • Almost all have chronic sinusitis • CXR and HRCT show diffuse small centrilobular nodular opacities and hyperinflation

Classification of COPD by severity

Stage 0: At risk	Lung function still normal (normal spirometry); chronic symptoms (chronic cough and sputum production)
Stage I: Mild COPD	Mild airflow limitation ($FEV_1/FVC < 70\%$ but $FEV1 \geq 80\%$ predicted) and usually, but not always, chronic cough and sputum production • *At this stage, the individual may not be aware that his or her lung function is abnormal*
Stage II: Moderate COPD	Worsening airflow limitation ($FEV_1/FVC < 70\%$, $50\% \leq FEV_1 < 80\%$ predicted) and usually progression of symptoms, with shortness of breath typically developing on exertion
Stage III: Severe COPD	Further worsening of airflow limitation ($FEV1/FVC < 70\%$, $30\% \leq FEV_1 < 50\%$ predicted), ↑ shortness of breath and repeated exacerbations which have impact on patient's quality of life
Stage IV: Very severe COPD	Severe airflow limitation ($FEV_1/FVC < 70\%$, $FEV_1 < 30\%$ predicted) or $FEV_1 < 50\%$ plus chronic respiratory failure • *At this stage, quality of life is very appreciably impaired and exacerbations may be life-threatening*

Global Initiative for Chronic Obstructive Lung Disease (GOLD), Executive Summary: Global strategy for the diagnosis, management and prevention of COPD, updated September 2005. (Based on April 1998 NHLBI/WHO Workshop) www.goldcopd.com

8.3.2   Component 2: Reduce risk factors

Smoking cessation

Single most effective and cost-effective way to reduce the risk of developing COPD and stop its progression (does NOT reverse damage)

Strategy to Help a Patient Quit Smoking

1. **ASK**: Systematically identify all tobacco users at every visit.
Implement an office-wide system that ensures that, for EVERY patient at EVERY clinic visit, tobacco-use status is queried and documented.

2. **ADVISE**: Strongly urge all tobacco users to quit.
In a clear, strong and personalized manner, urge every tobacco user to quit.

3. **ASSESS**: Determine willingness to make a quit attempt.
Ask every tobacco user if he or she is willing to make a quit attempt at this time (e.g., within the next 30 days).

4. **ASSIST**: Aid the patient in quitting.
Help the patient with a quit plan; provide practical counseling; provide intra-treatment social support; help the patient obtain extra-treatment social support; recommend use of approved pharmacotherapy if appropriate; provide supplementary materials.

5. **ARRANGE**: Schedule follow-up contact.
Schedule follow-up contact, either in person or via telephone.

Global Initiative for Chronic Obstructive Lung Disease (GOLD), Executive Summary: Global strategy for the diagnosis, management and prevention of COPD, updated September 2005. (Based on April 1998 NHLBI/WHO Workshop) www.goldcopd.com

Pharmacotherapy

- **Nicotine replacement therapy:** in any form (e.g. nicotine gum, inhaler, sublingual tablet, nasal spray, transdermal patch) increases long-term smoking quit rates
- **Antidepressants: bupropion** (Zyban) and **nortriptyline** also increase long-term quit rates

Occupational exposures

Eliminate, reduce and/or control occupational exposure to inhaled particles and gases

Indoor/outdoor air pollution

Implement measures to decrease and/or avoid indoor air and outdoor air pollution. Advise patients to monitor public announcements for air quality

8.3.3   Component 3: Managing stable COPD

Pharmacologic treatment (see table below)

- **Bronchodilators**
  - Give "as-needed" to relieve intermittent or worsening symptoms and on a regular basis to prevent or reduce persistent symptoms
  - The choice between β_2 agonists, anticholinergics, methylxanthines and combination therapy depends on availability of medications and patient's response (e.g. symptom relief and side effects)
  - Regular treatment with long-acting bronchodilators is more effective and convenient than treatment with short-acting bronchodilators, but more expensive
  - Combining drugs with different mechanisms and durations of action may increase the degree of bronchodilation for equivalent or lesser side effects
  - Theophylline is effective in COPD, but due to its potential toxicity, inhaled bronchodilators are preferred when available

- **Glucocorticosteroids**
  - Regular treatment with inhaled glucocorticosteroids is appropriate for symptomatic patients with FEV_1 < 50% of predicted (Stage III: severe COPD and Stage IV: very severe COPD) and repeated exacerbations (e.g. 3 exacerbations in the last 3 years)
  - Prolonged treatment with inhaled glucocorticosteroids may relieve symptoms in this carefully selected group of patients but does not modify the long-term decline in FEV1. The dose-response relationships and long-term safety of inhaled glucocorticosteroids in COPD are not known. Long-term treatment with oral glucocorticosteroids is not recommended

Commonly used formulations of Drugs for COPD					
Drug	Inhaler (mg)	Solution for nebulizer (mg/ml)	Oral	Vials for injection (mg)	Duration of action (hours)
β2 agonists: short-acting					
Fenoterol**	100 - 200 (MDI)	1	0.05%		(syrup) 4 - 6
Salbutamol (Albuterol)	100, 200 (MDI & DPI)	5	5 mg (pill) Syrup (0.024%)	0.1, 0.5	4 - 6
Terbutaline	400, 500 (DPI)	-	2.5, 5 (pill)	0.2, 0.25	4 - 6
β_2 agonists: long-acting					
Formoterol	4.5 - 12 (MDI & DPI)				12 +
Salmeterol	25 - 50 (MDI & DPI)				12 +
Anticholinergics: short-acting					
Ipratropium bromide	20, 40 (MDI)	0.25 - 0.5			6 - 8
Oxitropium bromide**	100 (MDI)	1.5			7 - 9
Anticholinergics: long-acting					
Tiotropium	18 (DPI)				24 +
Combination: short-acting β_2 agonist plus anticholinergic in one inhaler					
Fenoterol/ Ipratropium	200/80 (MDI)	1.25/0.5			6 - 8
Salbutamol/ Ipratropium	75/15 (MDI)	0.75/4.5			6 - 8

Methylxanthines					
Aminophylline			200 – 600 mg (pill)	240 mg	Variable, up to 24 h
Theophylline (SR)			100 – 600 mg (pill)		Variable, up to 24 h
Inhaled glucocorticosteroids					
Beclomethasone	50 – 400 (MDI & DPI)	0.2 – 0.4			
Budesonide	100, 200, 400 (DPI)	0.20, 0.25, 0.5			
Fluticasone	50 – 500 (MDI & DPI)				
Triamcinolone	100 (MDI)	40		40	
Combination: long–acting β2 agonists plus glucocorticosteroids in one inhaler					
Formoterol/ Budesonide**	4.5/80, 160 (DPI) (9/320) (DPI)				
Salmeterol/ Fluticasone	50/100, 250, 500 (DPI) 25/50, 125, 250 (MDI)				
Systemic glucocorticosteroids					
Prednisone			5 – 60 mg (pill)		
Methyl- prednisolone	10 – 2000 mg		4, 8, 16 mg (pill)		

Key: ** = available outside of US;
MDI = metered dose inhaler; DPI = dry powder inhaler

Global Initiative for Chronic Obstructive Lung Disease (GOLD), Executive Summary: Global Strategy for the Diagnosis, Management and Prevention of COPD, updated September 2005. (Based on April 1998 NHLBI/WHO Workshop) www.goldcopd.com

- **Other pharmacologic treatments**
  - **Vaccines:** Influenza vaccines can ↓ serious illness and death in COPD by ~ 50%. Should be given once (in autumn) or twice (in autumn and winter) each year. Pneumococcal vaccine has been used but more evidence is needed to support its general use in COPD patients
  - **Alpha-1 antitrypsin augmentation therapy:** young patients with severe hereditary α-1 antitrypsin deficiency with established emphysema may be candidates; however, it is very expensive and is not available in most countries
  - **Antibiotics:** only for infectious exacerbations of COPD
  - **Mucolytics:** few patients with viscous sputum may benefit from mucolytics. Not recommended for widespread use
  - **NOT recommended for stable COPD:** regular use of antitussives, respiratory stimulants, narcotics, immunoregulators, antioxidants, nedocromil, leukotriene modifiers and alternative healing methods (e.g. herbal medicine, acupuncture and homeopathy). Vasodilators (e.g. inhaled NO) are contraindicated

Non-pharmacologic treatment
- **Pulmonary rehabilitation:** the goal is to reduce symptoms, improve quality of life and ↑ physical and emotional participation in daily activities. Patients at all stages of disease benefit from exercise training programs, with improvements in exercise tolerance and symptoms of dyspnea and fatigue. The longer the program continues, the more effective the results.
- **Oxygen therapy:**
  - Long-term O_2 therapy (> 15 hours per day) is usually introduced in Stage IV: very severe COPD, for patients who have:
    - PaO_2 < 55 mmHg (7.3 kPa) or SaO_2 ≤ 88% with or without hypercapnia; **or**
    - PaO_2 55 - 60 mmHg (7.3 - 8.0 kPa) or SaO_2 89% with evidence of pH, peripheral edema suggesting CHF or polycythemia (Hct > 55%)
  - The goal of long-term oxygen therapy is PaO_2 of at least 60 mmHg (8.0 kPa) at sea level and rest and/or SaO_2 ≥ 90%
- **Surgical interventions:**
  - **Bullectomy:** in carefully selected patients (of grad IV of COPD), effective in reducing dyspnea and improving lung function
  - **Lung volume reduction surgery (LVRS):** still unproven palliative procedure; not recommended if FEV_1 < 20% and either homogeneous emphysema on HRCT or D_LCO < 20%

○ **Lung transplantation:** may be considered in carefully selected patients with advanced COPD (Stage IV: very severe COPD); may improve quality of life and functional capacity; criteria for lung transplantation include: $FEV_1 < 35\%$ predicted, $PaO_2 < 55 - 60$ mmHg (7.3 - 8.0 kPa), $PaCO_2 > 50$ mmHg (> 6.7 kPa) and secondary PH

Surgical options for COPD patients

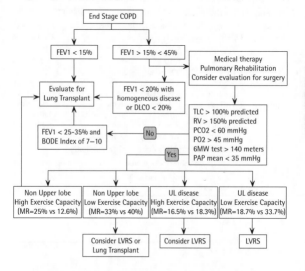

TLC = total lung capacity; RV = residual volume; 6MW test = 6-min walk test; UL disease = upper-lobe-predominant disease; Non Upper lobe = non-upper-lobe disease distribution; MR = mortality rates. Comparisons of LVRS vs medical therapy in each of the four groups were made with a median follow-up period of 29 months.

Fig. 20 Suggested algorithm of surgical options for COPD patients
Modified from/source: Nathan, Steven D., CHEST 2005; 127: 1006-1016.

NOTE: *There is no convincing evidence that mechanical ventilation has a role in routine management of stable COPD.*

But non invasive ventilation may be of benfit in a selected group of patients. It´s efficacious in acute exacerbation of COPD with acute respiratory failure in reducing mortality, reducing the klength of hospital stay and preventing intubation (s. 8.3.4).

GOLD severity staging of COPD and recommended treatment

Classification of Severity* (stages 0 - IV) and characteristics of COPD

0: At risk	I: Mild COPD	II: Moderate COPD	III: Severe COPD	IV: Very severe COPD
• Normal spirometry • Exposure to risk factors • Chronic symptoms[a]	• FEV_1/FVC < 70% • FEV_1 ≥ 80% predicted • With or without chronic symptoms[a]	• FEV_1/FVC < 70% • 50% ≤ FEV_1 < 80% predicted • With or without chronic symptoms[a]	• FEV_1/FVC < 70% • 30% ≤ FEV_1 < 50% predicted • With or without chronic symptoms[a]	• FEV_1/FVC < 70% • FEV_1 < 30% predicted or respiratory failure[b] or right heart failure
Avoidance of risk factors; influenza vaccination				
	Add short-acting bronchodilator when needed			
		Add regular treatment with one or more long-acting bronchodilators; **Add** rehabilitation		
			Add inhaled glucocorticosteroids if repeated exacerbations	
				Add long-term O_2 if chronic respiratory failure; **Consider** surgical treatments

*: classification is based on postbronchodilator FEV_1
a: cough, sputum production
b: respiratory failure: PaO_2 < 60 mmHg with or without $PaCO_2$ > 50 mmHg while breathing room air at sea level

Global Initiative for Chronic Obstructive Lung Disease (GOLD), Executive Summary:
Global Strategy for the Diagnosis, Management and Prevention of COPD, updated September 2005. (Based on April 1998 NHLBI/WHO Workshop) www.goldcopd.com

8.3.4 Component 4: Manage exacerbations

The most common causes of an exacerbation of COPD are infection of the tracheobronchial tree or air pollution. The cause of ~ $\frac{1}{3}$ of severe exacerbation cannot be identified.

Diagnosis and assessment of severity
Indicators of COPD exacerbation:
- Increased breathlessness, wheezing, chest tightness, increased cough and sputum, change of color ± tenacity of sputum and fever
- **Pulmonary function tests (PFT):** may be difficult for sick patient to perform
  - PEF < 100 L/min or FEV_1 < 1 L indicates severe exacerbation
- **Arterial blood gases (ABG)** in hospital: PaO_2 < 60 mmHg (< 8.0 kPa) and/or SaO_2 < 90% with or without $PaCO_2$ > 50 mmHg (> 6.7 kPa) when breathing room air indicates respiratory failure; PaO_2 < 6.7 kPa (50 mm Hg), $PaCO2$ > 9.3 kPa (70 mm Hg) and pH < 7.30 suggest a life-threatening episode that needs close monitoring or critical management
- **Chest X-ray:** posterior/anterior plus lateral identify conditions such as pneumonia and alternative diagnoses that may mimic symptoms of COPD exacerbations
- **ECG:** helps in diagnosis of right ventricular hypertrophy, arrhythmias and ischemic episodes
- **Other laboratory tests:** when an infectious exacerbation does not respond to initial antibiotic therapy, a sputum culture and antibiogram should be performed. Biochemical tests may help identify wether the cause of an exacerbation is an electrolyte imbalance, diabetes or poor nutrition

Home management
- **Bronchodilators:** the dose and/or frequency of existing bronchodilator therapy should be increased and if not already used, an anticholinergic should be added until symptoms improve

- **Glucocorticosteroids:** if baseline FEV_1 < 50% predicted, consider adding prednisolone 40 mg/day (PO) for 10 days to bronchodilators. Nebulized budesonide may be an alternative to oral glucocorticosteroids for nonacidotic exacerbations
- **Antibiotics:** only effective when patients with worsening dyspnea and cough also have increased sputum volume and purulence. Take into account local patterns of antibiotic sensitivity when choosing antibiotic agent

Hospital management

Indications for hospital assessment or admission for exacerbations of COPD:
- Marked ↑ in intensity of symptoms (e.g. sudden onset of resting dyspnea)
- Severe background COPD
- Onset of new physical signs (e.g. cyanosis, peripheral edema)
- Failure of exacerbation to respond to initial medical therapy
- Significant comorbidities
- New arrhythmias
- Older age and/or insufficient home support

Indications for ICU Admission:
- Severe dyspnea not responding adequately to initial therapy
- Confusion, lethargy, coma
- Persistent or worsening hypoxemia (PaO_2 < 40 mmHg, < 5.3 kPa) and/or
- Severe/worsening hypercapnia ($PaCO_2$ > 60 mmHg, > 8.0 kPa) and/or severe worsening respiratory acidosis (pH < 7.25), despite supplemental O_2 and NIPPV

Management of severe non-life threatening exacerbation of COPD in the emergency department or hospital:
- Assess severity of symptoms, blood gases, CXR
- **Controlled O_2 therapy** to achieve PaO_2> 60 mmHg (> 8.0 kPa) or SaO_2 > 90%
- Venturi masks are more accurate source of controlled O_2 than nasal cannula, but are less comfortable and may be removed by the patient
- Obtain ABG 30 min after initiating O_2 therapy to ensure satisfactory oxygenation without CO_2 retention or acidosis
- **Bronchodilators:** short-acting inhaled β_2 agonists are usually preferred for exacerbation of COPD. Increase dose or frequency if necessary to
- Add an **anticholinergic** to short-acting β_2 agonist if there is no prompt response to β_2 agonist
- Consider adding **methylxanthine** (PO or IV) for more severe exacerbations. Must monitor serum theophylline levels to avoid side effects

- **Glucocorticosteroids**: oral or IV glucocorticosteroids are recommended as an addition to bronchodilator therapy. Exact dose that should be given is not known, but high doses $\Rightarrow \uparrow$ risk of side effects
- **Prednisolone** 30 - 40 mg PO for 10 - 14 days is reasonable
- Antibiotics: only effective when patients with worsening dyspnea and cough also have $\uparrow$ sputum volume and purulence. Take into account local patterns of antibiotic sensitivity when choosing antibiotic agent

Stratification of patients with COPD exacerbated for antibiotic treatment and potential microorganisms involved in each group

Goup[a]	Definition[b]	Microorganisms
Group A: Patients not requiring hospitalization (Stage I: Mild COPD)	Mild exacerbation	H. influenzae; S. pneumoniae M. catarrhalis; Chlamydia pneumoniae[c]; Viruses
Group B: Patients admitted to hospital (Stages II-IV: Moderate to Very Severe COPD)	Moderate-severe exacerbation without risk factors for P. aeruginosa infection	Group A plus: Enterobacteriaceae (K. pneumoniae, E. coli, Proteus, Enterobacter, etc)
Group C: Patients admitted to hospital (Stages II-IV: Moderate to Very Severe COPD)	Moderate-severe exacerbation with risk factors for P. aeruginosa infection	Group B plus: P. aeruginosa

a. In some settings, patients with moderate to severe exacerbation may be treated as outpatients. In this case, patients may best be stratified into two groups: an uncomplicated group without any risk factors and a complicated group that has one or more 'risk factors' (co-morbidity, severe COPD, frequent exacerbations, antimicrobial use within 3 months). The uncomplicated group: use Group A recommendations of 'Antibiotic treatment in exacerbations of COPD'. Complicated group: use Group B or C recommendations of 'Antibiotic treatment in exacerbations of COPD'.

b. Severity refers to the exacerbation, though this is interwindes with the severity of the underlying condition.

c. Chlamydia pneumonia (or Chlamidophila pneumoniae) has not been confirmed as a cause of exacerbations in some areas (e.g., UK).

Global Initiative for Chronic Obstructive Lung Disease (GOLD), Executive Summary: Global strategy for the diagnosis, management and prevention of COPD, updated September 2005. (Based on April 1998 NHLBI/WHO Workshop) www.goldcopd.com

Antibiotic treatment in exacerbations of COPD [a,b]

	Oral Treatment (no particular order)	Alternative (no particular order)	Parental Treatment (no particular order)
Group A	Patients with only one cardinal symptom should not receive antibiotics If indication then: • β-lactam (Ampicillin/ Amoxicillin[c]) • Tetracycline • Trimethoprim/ Sulfamethoxazole	• β-lactam/β-lactamase inhibitor (Co-amoxiclav) • Macrolides (Azithromycin, Clarithromycin, Roxithromycin[d]) • Cephalosporins - 2nd or 3rd generation • Ketolides (Telithromycin)	
Group B	• β-lactam/ β-lactamase inhibitor (Co-amoxiclav)	• Fluoroquinolones[d] (Gatifloxacin, Gemi-floxacin, Levofloxacin, Moxifloxacin)	• β-lactam/β- lactamase inhibitor (Co-amoxiclav, Ampicillin/ Sulbactam) • Cephalosporins - 2nd or 3rd generation • Fluoroquinolones[d] (Gatifloxacin, Levofloxacin, Moxifloxacin)

Group C	• Fluoroquinolones (Ciprofloxacin, Levofloxacin - high dose[e])	• Fluoroquinolones (Ciprofloxacin, Levofloxacin - high dose[e]) or • β-lactam with *P.aeruginosa* activity

a. All patients with symptoms of a COPD exacerbation should be treated with additional bronchodilators ± glucocorticosteroids.

b. Classes of antibiotics are provided (with specific agents in parentheses). In countries with high incidence of *S. pneumoniae* resistant to penicillin, high dosages of Amoxicillin or Co-Amoxiclav are recommended. (See 'Stratification of patients with COPD exacerbated for antibiotic treatment and potential' for definition of Groups A, B, C.)

c. This antibiotic is not appropriate in areas where there is increased prevalence of β-lactamase producing *H. influenzae* and *M. catarrhalis* and/or of *S. pneumoniae* resistant to penicillin.

d. Not available in all areas of the world.

e. Dose 750 mgs effective against *P. aeruginosa*.

Global Initiative for Chronic Obstructive Lung Disease (GOLD), Executive Summary: Global strategy for the diagnosis, management and prevention of COPD, updated September 2005. (Based on April 1998 NHLBI/WHO Workshop) www.goldcopd.com

- **Ventilatory support:**
  - **Noninvasive positive pressure ventilation (NIPPV)**
    Selection criteria:
    - Moderate-to-severe dyspnea with use of accessory muscles and paradoxical abdominal motion
    - pH < 7.35 and $PaCO_2$ > 45 mmHg, > 6.0 kPa
    - Respiratory rate > 25/min
    Exclusion criteria:
    - Respiratory arrest
    - Cardiovascular instability (hypotension, arrhythmias, MI)
    - Somnolence, impaired mental status and/or uncooperative patient
    - High risk for aspiration; viscous or copious secretions
    - Recent facial or gastroesophageal surgery
    - Craniofacial trauma, fixed nasopharyngeal abnormalities
    - Extreme obesity

- ○ **Invasive positive pressure ventilation (IPPV)**
  Indications:
    - Severe dyspnea with use of accessory muscles and paradoxical abdominal motion
    - Respiratory rate> 35/min
    - Life-threatening hypoxemia
      ($PaO_2 < 40$ mmHg, < 5.3 kPa or $PaO_2/FIO_2 < 200$)
    - pH < 7.25 and $PaCO_2 > 60$ mmHg, > 8.0 kPa
    - Respiratory arrest
    - Somnolence, impaired mental status
    - Cardiovascular complications (hypotension, shock, heart failure)
    - Other complications (metabolic abnormalities, sepsis, pneumonia, pulmonary embolism, barotraumas, massive pleural effusion)
    - NIPPV failure or exclusion criteria

- **Other measures:**
  - ○ Fluid administration (monitor fluid balance)
  - ○ Supplemental nutrition when too dyspneic to eat
  - ○ Low molecular weight heparin for immobilized, polycythemic or dehydrated patients with or without history of thromboembolic disease
  - ○ Sputum clearance by stimulating coughing and forced expirations
  - ○ Chest percussion and postural drainage may be beneficial in patients producing > 25 ml sputum/day or with lobar atelectasis

Discharge criteria for patients with exacerbations of COPD
- Inhaled β2-agonist therapy is required no more frequently than every 4 hrs
- Patient, if previously ambulatory, is able to walk across room
- Patient is able to eat and sleep without frequent awakening by dyspnea
- Patient has been clinically stable for 12-24 hrs
- Arterial blood gases have been stable for 12-24 hrs
- Patient (or home caregiver) fully understands correct use of medications
- Follow-up and home care arrangements have been completed (e.g., visiting nurse, oxygen delivery, meal provisions)
- Patient, family, and physician are confident patient can manage successfully

Follow-up assessment 4-6 weeks after discharge from hospital for exacerbations of COPD
- Ability to cope in usual environment
- Measurement of FEV1

- Reassessment of inhaler technique
- Understanding of recommended treatment regimen
- Need for long-term oxygen therapy and/or home nebulizer (for patients with very severe COPD)

Global Initiative for Chronic Obstructive Lung Disease (GOLD), Executive Summary: Global Strategy for the Diagnosis, Management and Prevention of COPD, updated September 2005. (Based on April 1998 NHLBI/WHO Workshop) www.goldcopd.com

8.4 Bronchiectasis

Definition

Irreversible dilatation of bronchi ± bronchioles secondary to destruction of airway walls (destruction of elastic and muscular components of bronchial wall). Often undiagnosed: persons with chronic sputum production are usually assumed to have chronic bronchitis

Classification

Cylindrical:
Dilated bronchial walls. Least severe type. Often bilateral and at the lower (dorsobasal) lobes

Fusiform:
Dilated bronchi have terminal bulbous enlargements

Saccular:
Full destruction of bronchial walls. Normal tissue is replaced by fibrotic tissue. This is the most severe type of bronchiectasis. Often diffuse.

Etiology

- Chronic (recurrent) infections
- Kartagener's syndrome (bronchiectasis, sinusitis, dextrocardia): immotile cilia (ciliary dyskinesia)
- Associated with cystic fibrosis, pulmonary tuberculosis, bronchial obstruction (tumor, enlarged hilar lymph nodes or aspirated objects), allergic bronchopulmonary aspergillosis, foreign body aspiration

Pathophysiology

- Because of bronchial wall destruction, mucociliary mechanism is impaired, which results in accumulation of large amounts of foul smelling secretions. Retained secretions promote infection and inflammation

- Small bronchi and bronchioles distal to affected area become obstructed with secretions, which leads to: (1) hyperinflation of distal alveoli as a result of inability of alveoli to expel air on expiration and/or (2) atelectasis or consolidation

Clinical manifestations
- Productive chronic cough with large amounts of purulent secretions
- Recurrent infections
- Dyspnea, hemoptysis (common), rhonchi and moist crackles, possibly wheezing, and digital clubbing
- Hypoxemia/hypercapnia if large area involved
- Sputum separates in 3 layers if left standing: upper layer is frothy and watery, middle layer is mucopurulent and bottom layer is opaque and purulent and may contain abscess material
- PFT = ↓ FVC, ↓ FEV_1, ↑ RV

Complications
- Brain abscess, amyloidosis
- Respiratory insufficiency, cor pulmonale
- Hemoptysis
- Aspergilloma
- Infection with Mycobacterium avium complex

Diagnosis
- **Chest X-ray:** linear atelectasis, dilated and thickened airways (tram or parallel lines), irregular peripheral opacities (sign of mucopurulent plaques)
- **CT scan** of 1 - 2 mm slices; CT scanning has replaced bronchography as the diagnostic gold standard
- **Bronchography:** old method which can still be used if CT scan is unavailable

Treatment
- Antibiotics to prevent and control recurrent infections, in the early phase of illness with *Streptococcus pneumoniae* and *Haemophilus* and later with Gram-negative spectrum, especially *Pseudomonas*. Also, antibiotics are also given via aerosol therapy (e.g. gentamicin, tobramicin)
- Bronchial hygiene therapy: chest physiotherapy (CPT), aerosol therapy, postural drainage
- Bronchodilators for airway obstruction
- O_2 for hypoxemia
- Surgical resection if bronchiectasis is limited to one lobe
- Pneumococcal and annual flu vaccine

9. Acute Respiratory Distress Syndrome (ARDS)

Definition
- Acute, diffuse parenchymal disease resulting in pulmonary (non-cardiogenic) edema and refractory hypoxemia secondary to injury of A-C membrane
- Defined clinically as acute lung illness characterized by development of bilateral lung infiltrates on CXR and severe hypoxemia ($PaO_2/FIO_2 < 200$) in the absence of CHF. Definition of acute lung injury (ALI): $PaO_2/FIO_2 < 300$

Etiology
- ARDS generally occurs in patients who are already weakened by illness
- Some causes of ARDS include: aspiration (gastric contents, toxic material), sepsis, shock, near drowning, trauma, prolonged high FIO_2, inhalational injury, blood transfusions and many more known and unknown causes

Pathophysiology
- ARDS is a complication that is caused by conditions that activate inflammatory mediators; this results in diffuse parenchymal lung injury, non-cardiogenic pulmonary edema and damage to pulmonary vasculature
- During the acute phase of ARDS, inflammatory cells release mediators which damage the integrity of the A-C membrane and ↑ permeability ⇒ pulmonary edema
- ↓ Surfactant production, loss of functioning alveoli and ↑ V/Q mismatch ⇒ refractory hypoxemia and respiratory failure
- Hyaline membranes form during subsequent healing phase

Clinical manifestations
- Refractory hypoxemia and possibly cyanosis
- Signs include tachycardia, tachypnea and inspiratory crackles
- ↓ CL (stiff lungs) results in higher ventilatory pressures
- ↑ A - a gradient indicates shunting
- CXR shows diffuse infiltrates (honeycomb), increased opacity

Diagnosis
Internationally recognized criteria for diagnosis of ARDS are:
- Diffuse bilateral infiltrates on CXR
- No evidence of CHF (pulmonary artery wedge pressure [PAWP] < 18 mmHg)
- Severe hypoxemia indicated by $PaO_2/FIO_2 < 200$; acute lung injury (ALI) = $PaO_2/FIO_2 < 300$

Treatment

First:
- Establish and treat the underlying cause
- Antibiotics for infections

Respiratory support:
- Mechanical ventilation with PEEP and FIO_2 to maintain adequate oxygenation: $PaO_2 > 60$ mmHg if possible; titrate PEEP to ↓ $FIO_2 < 0.50$ if possible. Use V_T of ~ 5 - 6 ml/kg ('low tidal volume ventilation'). Plateau pressure < 30 cmH_2O ± permissive hypercapnia
- Other aspects of respiratory support include pulmonary toilet, patient turning (prone position) and aspiration protection

Cardiovascular support:
- Inotropes may help maintain cardiac output and oxygen delivery
- Pulmonary vasodilators and fluid management should also be taken into consideration
- Diuretics may be prescribed to reduce interstitial edema

Other experimental therapies:
- High frequency ventilation?
- Extracorporeal membrane oxygenation (ECMO)?
- Surfactant replacement?
- Steroids?
  (Steroids such as methylprednisolone may help stabilize/suppress inflammation)
- Inhaled nitric oxide (iNO)

Prognosis
- Mortality 35 - 40% (has improved over the course of several years)
- Respiratory failure itself is unusual as a cause of death; complications such as nosocomial pneumonia and sepsis account for most deaths

10. Pulmonary Infections

10.1 Pneumonia

Definition

Infection of lung parenchyma (distal to terminal bronchiole), which leads to inflammation and exudates ⇒ air spaces filled with fluid (consolidation). This leads to reduced lung compliance and V/Q mismatch or shunt, which results in decreased oxygenation. Pneumonia is the 6th leading cause of death in the USA.

10.1.1 Community-acquired pneumonia (CAP)

Definition

Pneumonia acquired outside the hospital; common in nonimmuno-compromised individuals
Incidence ~ 2 - 4 million cases/year in the USA, with ~ 500,000 admissions (mortality ~ 10% [45,000]). ~ 25% of CAP cases require hospitalization

Etiology

Microbial agent	% cases	Microbial agent	% cases
BACTERIA		ATYPICAL	2 - 10
Streptococcus pneumoniae[1]	20 - 60	*Legionella*	2 - 8
Haemophilus influenzae	3 - 10	*Mycoplasma pneumoniae*	1 - 6
Staphylococcus aureus	3 - 5	*Chlamydia pneumoniae*	4 - 6
Gram (-) bacilli: *Klebsiella pneumoniae* *Acinetobacter* *Pseudomonas aeruginosa*	3 - 10	VIRAL[2] Influenza A (most common) *Parainfluenza Respiratory syncytial virus* (RSV; most common in children)	2 - 15
Miscellaneous: *Moraxella catarrhalis*, *Acinetobacter*	3 - 5	ASPIRATION pneumonia UNKNOWN	6 - 10 30 - 60

* Bartlett JG, Mundy LM: Community-acquired Pneumonia, N Engl J Med 1995; 333: 1616-1624.

1. Associated with bacteremia in 20 - 30% of cases,
2. ~ 90% of childhood pneumonia is viral

Clinical features

- Fever (bacterial)
- Chills
- Pleuritic chest pain
- Leukocytosis (bacterial)
- Dyspnea
- ± Pleural friction rub
- Productive cough
- Crackles over affected area
- Dullness to percussion
- Bronchial breath sounds
- Hypoxemia ± cyanosis
- Tachycardia/tachypnea
- CXR: lobar or segmental consolidation; diffuse alveolar or interstitial infiltrates (opacification)
- PFTs: restrictive pattern
- ↓ BS on affected side

Decision to hospitalize

The following risk factors are associated with increased mortality or the risk of a complicated course for CAP. These predictions/rules are intended to support, rather than replace, physician-guided decision-making.

Predicting Risks from CAP

(Fine MJ et al: N Engl J Med, 1997; 336: 243-250)

STEP I

Is patient > 50 years old?		
⇓ NO	YES ⇒	Assign patient to risk class II - V (step II below)
Does patient have history of any of the following comorbidities?		
• Neoplastic, renal or liver disease • CHF • Cerebrovascular disease		
⇓ NO	YES ⇒	
Does patient have any of the following examination findings?		
• Altered level of consciousness • HR ≥ 125 beats/min • RR ≥ 30/min • sysBP < 90 mmHg • Temp < 35 or ≥ 40°C		
⇓ NO	YES ⇒	
Patient is in risk class I (low risk)		

STEP II
see next page

STEP II

PORT Scoring System for Hospitalization of Community-Acquired Pneumonia

Patient characteristic	Points
Demographics	
Men	Age in years
Women	Age −10
Nursing home resident	+ 10
Comorbid illness	
Malignancy	+ 30
Liver disease	+ 20
Congestive heart failure	+ 10
Cerebrovascular disease	+ 10
Renal disease	+ 10
Physical examination	
Altered mental status	+ 20
Resp rate ≥ 30/min	+ 20
sysBP < 90 mmHg	+ 20
Temp. < 35 or ≥ 40°C	+ 15
HR ≥ 125 beats/min	+ 10
Laboratory/CXR	
pH < 7.35	+ 30
BUN ≥ 30 mg/dl	+ 20
Na^+ < 130 mmol/L	+ 20
Glucose ≥ 250 mg/d	+ 10
Hct < 30%	+ 10
PaO_2 < 60 mmHg	+ 10
Pleural effusion	+ 10

Stratification of risk factors		
Total Points	Risk Class	Hospitalize
None (see step I)	I	No
< 70	II	No

NOTE: *Other risk factors include: old age (> 65 years), cigarette smoking, COPD, alcoholism, HIV infection, steroid therapy, history of pneumonia, poor dental hygiene, IV drug use, creatinine > 1.2 mg/dl, extrapulmonary site of infection, neurologic disorders, leukopenia (< 4000 WBC/mm^3) or leukocytosis (> 20,000 WBC/mm^3), CXR shows > 1 lobe involvement, cavity and/or pleural effusion and Hb < 9 g/dl.*

Diagnosis

- Clinical presentation; consider when newly acquired: cough, sputum production, dyspnea, fever, abnormal breath sounds (bronchial and/or localized crackles), tachypnea
- CXR: new infiltrates; all patients with CAP should have CXR to establish Diagnosis and any presence of complications (pleural effusion, multilobar disease)
- Sputum Gram's stain and culture
  - Properly collected expectorated sputum is helpful for focusing initial empiric therapy
  - If used, should have > 25 WBCs and < 10 squamous cells/low powered field
- Blood culture x 2 before antibiotic treatment
- Bronchoscopy with protected brush catheter or bronchoalveolar lavage (BAL): consider for severely ill and failure to respond to treatment
- Acid-fast bacillus (AFB) culture and sensitivity with cough > 1 month and < 1 year
- Serology is not helpful
- With severe CAP, Legionella urinary antigen assay test (especially in endemic areas)
- Thoracentesis should be performed when > 1 cm of fluid on a lateral decubitus film
  - Studies: lactate dehydrogenase (LDH), cell count and differential, protein, glucose, pH culture and sensitivity

Treatment

American Thoracic Society (ATS) recommendations are summarized below. ~ 80% of all CAP cases are managed in outpatient clinics, while ~ 20% of CAP patients are hospitalized. Antibiotic treatment is preferably specific, but is often initially empiric.

ATS recommended empiric therapy for community-aquired pneumonia

I. Outpatient CAP

No cardiopulmonary disease (e.g. CHF, COPD) and/or modifying risk factors	Macrolide antibiotics[a]: azithromycin **or** clarithromycin **or** Doxycycline (azithromycin and clarithromycin preferred over erythromycin if *H. influenzae* suspected)

II. Outpatient CAP

Cardiopulmonary disease (e.g. CHF, COPD) and/or other modifying risk factors	β-lactam[c]: cefpodoxime, cefuroxime, high-dose amoxicillin, amoxicillin-clavulanate **or** parenteral ceftriaxone followed by oral cefpodoxime + Macrolide or doxycycline **or** Antipneumococcal fluoroquinolone[b] alone

III. Inpatient CAP: non-ICU

Cardiopulmonary disease (e.g. CHF, COPD) and/or modifying risk factors (including living in a nursing home)	IV β-lactam: cefotaxime, ceftriaxone, ampicillin-sulbactam[d] **or** high-dose ampicillin + IV or PO macrolide: azithromycin, clarithromycin **or** doxycycline **or** IV antipneumococcal fluoroquinolone alone
No cardiopulmonary disease, no modifying risk factors	IV azithromycin alone **or** if macrolide allergic/intolerant: doxycycline + β-lactam **or** antipneumococcal fluoroquinolone alone

IV. Hospitalized: ICU

No risks for Pseudomonal aeruginosa	IV cefotaxime or ceftriaxone + IV azithromycin **or** IV fluoroquinolone
Risks for Pseudomonas aeruginosa	IV antipseudomonal β-lactam[e] + IV ciprofloxacin **or** IV antipseudomonal β-lactam + IV ciprofloxacin + IV azithromycin **or** IV nonpseudomonal quinolone

American Thoracic Society: Guidelines for the Management of Adults with Community-acquired Pneumonia: Diagnosis, Assessment of Severity, Antimicrobial Therapy and Prevention, Am J Respir Crit Care Med 2001; 163: 1730-1754.

Key:
a: Macrolide: azithromycin [Zithromax], clarithromycin [Biaxin], erythromycin
b: Fluoroquinolone: levofloxacin [Levaquin], gatifloxacin [Tequin], moxifloxacin [Avelox]
c: β-Lactam: cefotaxime [Claforan], ceftriaxone [Rocephin], cefpodoxime
d: β-Lactam/β-lactamase inhibitor: ampicillin/sulbactam [Unasyn], amoxicillin/clavulanate [Augmentin], piperacillin/tazobactam [Zosyn]
e: Antipseudomonal β-lactam: cefepime, imipenem, meropenem, piperacillin/tazobactam

Modifying factors that increase the risk for infection with specific pathogens

Penicillin and drug-resistant pneumococci	Enteric Gram-negative infections	Pseudomonas aeruginosa
• Age > 65 years • Alcoholism • β-lactam therapy in past 3 months • Multiple comorbidities • Immunosuppression: illness, steroids • Exposure to child in daycare center	• Nursing home resident • Underlying cardiopulmonary disease • Multiple comorbidities • Recent antibiotic use	• Structural lung disease (bronchiectasis) • Corticosteroid therapy (> 10 mg/d of prednisone) • Broad-spectrum antibiotic therapy use for > 7 d in past month • Malnutrition

Other considerations

Duration of Treatment	*S. pneumoniae* and other bacterial infections: ~ 7 - 10 days; *M. pneumoniae, C. pneumoniae, Legionella*: 10 - 14 days; Patients chronically treated with corticosteroids: ≥ 14 days
Clinical response	Most patients with CAP respond to therapy within 3 days; if failure to respond, consider: incorrect diagnosis; host failure; inappropriate antibiotic, dose or route of administration; unusual pathogen; superinfection or empyema
Switch to oral therapy when	Improved cough and dyspnea; afebrile (< 38°C) on 2 occasions 8 hours apart; decreasing WBC count toward normal; functioning GI tract with adequate oral intake (fluids, food, ± medications)
Discharge	**Prevention:** consider Pneumococcal, influenza vaccine upon discharge; encourage smoking cessation CXR: no need prior to discharge if patient clinically improving; consider CXR during follow-up office visit ~ 4 - 6 weeks after hospital discharge to get new X-ray baseline and to exclude any malignancies associated with CAP (especially in older smokers)

10.1.2 Hospital–acquired pneumonia (HAP)

Definition

(Nosocomial pneumonia) develops $\geq 48 - 72$ hours after hospital admission and is not apparent at admission. HAP is the 2nd most common hospital-acquired infection, but it has the highest mortality of all nosocomial infections.

Incidence

5 - 10 cases/1000 hospital admissions, but 6 - 20 times higher in patients receiving ventilatory support. HAP accounts for up to 25 percent of all ICU infections. HAP can be divided into:

(a) early onset HAP: occurs during 1st 4 days of hospitalization
(common pathogens: *S. pneumoniae*, methicillin-resistant *S. aureus* (MRSA), *H. influenzae*)

and

(b) late onset HAP: occurs after 4th day of hospitalization
(common pathogens: *S. aureus*, *P. aeruginosa*, *Acinetobacter*)

Routes of bacterial entry

- Aspiration (most common cause) of colonized oropharyngeal secretions or esophageal/gastric contents. Increased risk of aspiration: impaired gag reflex, altered level of consciousness (LOC) and use of ETT and/or NG tube
- Inhalation of infected aerosols (e.g. medication nebulizers, humidifiers)
- Exogenous penetration from infected site

Clinical features

- New or progressive pulmonary infiltrate on CXR
- Fever > 38.5 °C or hypothermia < 36 °C
- Leukocytosis > 12,000 WBC/mm^3 or leukopenia < 4000 WBC/mm^2
- Purulent secretions

Risk factors

- Intubated patient: prevention of cough reflex and compromised mucociliary clearance
- > 65 years of age
- Chronic lung disease
- Poor nutritional status
- Increased risk for aspiration (decreased LOC, intubated, tracheostomy, NG tube $\Rightarrow$ esophageal sphincter incompetence)

- Thoracic or upper abdomen surgery
- Altered host defenses (immunosuppressive therapy)
- Contaminated respiratory therapy equipment: resuscitation bags, humidifiers, medication nebulizers, stethoscopes
- Reintubation

Diagnosis

- Clinical: The presence of a new or progressive radiographic infiltrate plus at least two of three clinical features (fever greater than 38°C, leukocytosis or leukopenia, and purulent secretions) are most accurate for clinical diagnosis, in addition tachypnea, crackles, bronchial breath sounds
- Blood cultures x 2
- Pleural fluid culture with pleural effusion
- Gram's stain and cultures of lower reapiratory tract secretions (aspirated secretions or protective specimen-brushed secretions) bronchoscopic sampling if possible; if not available, sampling of reliable obtained lower respiratory tract secretions for quantitative cultures
- ABG: help define severity of HAP and need for oxygen

Treatment

Pathogen directed. Empiric treatment is often unnecessary, as Gram stain of respiratory secretions usually indicates probable pathogens and culture usually guides specific antibiotic selection.

Managemant strategies for patient with suspected hospital-aquiered pneumonia, ventilator-associated pneumonia, or healthcare-associated pneumonia

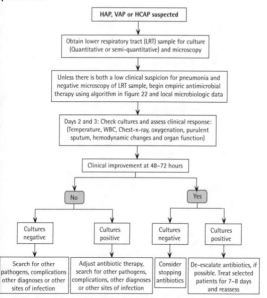

Fig. 21 Summary of the management strategies for a patient with suspected hospital-acquired pneumonia (HAP, ventilator-associated pneumonia (VAP), or healthcare-associated pneumonia (HCAP). The decision about antibiotic discontinuation may differ depending on the type of sample collected quantitative or semi quantitative terms.

Modified from/source: Guidelines for the Management of adults with hospital-aquired, Ventilator-associated, and Health-care associate Pneumonia. American Thoracic Society Documents. Am J Respir Crit Care Med 2005; 171:388.

Initiating empiric antibiotic therapy for hospital-aquiered pneumonia, ventilator-associated pneumonia, and healthcare-associated pneumonia

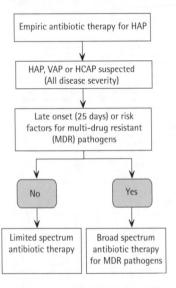

Fig. 22 Algorithm for initiating empiric antibiotic therapy for hospital-acquired pneumonia (HAP), ventilator-associated pneumonia (HCAP), and healthcare-associated pneumonia (HCAP).
Modified from/source: Guidelines for the Management of adults with hospital-acquired, Ventilator-associated, and Health-care associated Pneumonia. American Thoracic Society Documents. Am J Respir Crit Care Med 2005; 171:388.

Initial empiric antibiotic therapy for hospital-aquired pneumonia or ventilator-associated pneumonia in patients with no known risk factors for multidrug-resistant pathogens, early onset, and any disease severity

Potential pathogen	Recommended antibiotic*
Streptococcus pneumoniae**	Ceftriaxone
Hemophilus influenzae	or
Methicillin-sensitive Staphilococcus aureus	Levofloxacin, moxifloxacin, or ciprofloxacin
	or
Antibiotic-sensitive enteric gram-negative bacilli	Ampicillin/ sulbactam
Escherichia coli	or
Klebsiella pneumoniae	Ertapenem
Enterobacter species	
Proteus species	
Serratia marcescens	

*See table 'Initial Intravenous, Adult Doses of Antibiotics for Empiric Therapy of HAP, Including VAP, and HCAP in Patients with Late-Onset Disease or Risk Factors for Multidrug-Resistant Pathogens' for proper initial doses of antibiotics.

**The frequency of penicillin-resistant S.pneumoniae and mulidrug -resistant S.pneumoniae is increasing; levofloxacin or oxifloxacin are preferred to ciprofloxacin and the role of other new quinolones, such as gatifloxacin, has not been establisehd.

Guidelines for the Management of adults with hospital acquired, Ventilator-associated, and Health-care associated Pneumonia. American Thoracic Society Documents. Am J Respir Crit Care Med 2005; 171:388.

Initial empiric antibiotic therapy for hospital-acquired pneumonia or ventilator-associated pneumonia in patients with known risk factors for multidrug-resistant pathogens, early onset, and any disease severity

Potential pathogens	Combination antibiotic therapy*
Pathogens listed in previous table and MDR pathogens ○ *Pseudomonas aeruginosa* ○ *Klebsiella pneumoniae* (ESBL+)° ○ *Acinetobacter species*° ○ Methicillin-resistant *Staphilococcus aureus* (MRSA) *Legionella pneumophila*°	Antipseudomonal cephalosporin (cefepime, ceftazidime) or Antipseudomonal carbepenem (imipenem or meropenem) or β-Lactam / β-lactamase inhibitor (piperacillin-tazobactam) plus Antipseudomonal fluoroquinolone° (ciprofloxacin or levofloxacin) or Aminoglycoside (amikacin, gentamicin or tobramycin) plus Linezolid or vancomycin[+]

*See next table for adequate initial dosing of antibiotics. Initial antibiotic therapy should be adjusted or streamlined on the basis of microbiologic data and clinical response to therapy.
°If an ESBL strain, such as K. pneumoniae, or an Acinetobacter species is suspected, a carbepenem is a reliable choice. If L. pneumophila is suspected, the combination antibiotic regimen should include a macolide (e.g. azithromycin) or a fluoroquinolone (e.g. ciprofloxacin or levofloxacin) should be used rather than an aminoglycoside.
+If MRSA risk factors are present or there is a high incidence locally.

Guidelines for the Management of adults with hospital-acquired, Ventilator -associated and Health-care associate Pneumonia. American Thoracic Society Documents. Am J Respir Crit Care Med 2005; 171:388

Initial intravenous, adult doses of antibiotics for empiric therapy of hospital-acquired pneumonia, including ventilator-associated pneumonia, and healthcare-associated pneumonia in patients with late-onset disease or risk factors for multidrug-resistant pathogens

Antibiotic	Dosage*
Antipseudomonal cephalosporin	
• Cefepime	1-2g every 8-12h
• Ceftazidime	2g every 8h
Carbepenems	
• Imipenem	500mg every 6h or1g every 8h
• Meropenem	1g every 8h
β-Lactam/β-lactamase inhibitor	
• Piperacillin-tazobactam	4.5g every 6h
Aminoglycosides	
• Gentamicin	7mg/kg per d[+]
• Tobramycin	7mg/kg per d[+]
• Amikacin	20mg/kg per d[+]
Antipseudomonal quinolones	
• Levofloxacin	750mg every d
• Ciprofloxacin	400mg every 8h
Vancomycin	15mg/kg every 12h[++]
Linezolid	600mg every 12h

*Dosages are based on normal renal and hepatic function.
[+]Trough levels for gentamicin and tobramycin should be less than 1g/ml and for amikacin they should be less than 4-5g/ml.
[++]Tough levels for vancomycin should be 15-20g/ml.

Guidelines for the Management of adults with hospital acquired, Ventilator-associated, and Health-care associated Pneumonia. American Thoracic Society Documents. Am J Respir Crit Care Med 2005; 171:388.

Definition of severe HAP

Admission to ICU; respiratory failure: need for MV or > 35% O_2 for SaO_2 > 90%; rapid CXR progression, multilobar pneumonia or cavitation of lung infiltrate; evidence of sepsis with hypotension and/or end-organ dysfunction:

shock (sysBP < 90 mmHg or diaBP < 60 mmHg), need vasopressor for > 4 hours, urine output < 20 ml/h or < 80 ml in 4 h, acute renal failure requiring dialysis

Prevention

- Meticulous hand washing between each patient contact
- Isolating patients with highly resistant organisms, e.g. MRSA
- Keep patient semi-erect (> 30 - 45° angle) when feeding directly into stomach
- Continuous or intermittent subglottic suctioning above ETT cuff (requires special ETT that has second suction lumen located above cuff)
- Use heat and moisture exchanger (HME) instead of heated humidification during MV in adults, unless contraindicated
- Infrequent ventilator tubing changes: can be changed once/week or once/month or even between patients + PRN (no proof yet if any particular schedule reduces incidence of ventilator-associated pneumonia [VAP])
- ? Sucralfate instead of H_2 antagonist or antacids
- Postpyloric feeding if possible (not necessarily at day 1 after intubation)
- Glucose control (about 110mg/dl)
- Adequate disinfection of bronchoscopes
- Minimize sedation
- Use closed in-line suction catheters during MV

Recent study (JK Stoller et al: Respir Care 2003; 48(5): 494-499) showed that weekly vs the usual daily changing of in-line suction catheter does not appear to increase frequency of VAP.

(1) Ventilator associated pneumonia (VAP)

A subset of HAP. It is a complication of intubation and MV. VAP is defined as pneumonia occurring ≥ 24 hours after initiation of MV. Late-onset VAP: develops ≥ 96 hours after intubation. Early diagnosis of VAP is based on suspicion of new or progressing radiographic infiltrates.

(2) Aspiration pneumonia

Definition

Abnormal entry of oropharyngeal secretions or gastric contents or exogenous substances into lower airways. Chemical pneumonitis may be caused by aspiration of gastric acid, oil, meconium (newborns), noxious gases/smoke. Causes ≤ 15% of all CAP.

Predisposition

↑ risk for developing aspiration pneumonia

Decreased LOC	Anesthesia, drug OD, alcoholism, CVA, head trauma, NM disorders
Impaired mucociliary clearance	Cigarette smoking, ETT in place, ciliary dyskinesia
GI disorders	Protracted vomiting, gastric distention, sphincter incompetency, bowel obstruction, esophageal stricture
Mechanical barriers	ETT, TT, NG tube
Other	Dysphagia, gingivitis, periodontal disease, vocal cord disease

Clinical features

- Right lung is more involved than the left because the right main-stem bronchus forms a less acute angle (~ 20 - 30°) than the left main-stem bronchus, which forms 45 - 55° angle
- CXR: infiltrates in dependent lung lobes
- Tachypnea, fever, diffuse crackles, hypoxemia, productive cough with foul smelling sputum and ± bronchospasm with chemical pneumonitis

Treatment

- Clindamycin (450 - 900 mg IV q8h)
- Alternative:
  - Cefoxitin (2 mg IV 8 h)
  - Pipercillin [Zosyn] (3.375 g IV q6h)
  - Ticarcillin [Timentin] (3.1 g IV q6h)
- Supportive care:
  - O_2 for hypoxemia
  - Mechanical ventilation if needed
  - IV fluid support

Prevention: ↓ risk
- For patient with ETT/TT, ensure adequate cuff inflation pressure (25 - 35 cmH$_2$O)
- Raise HOB > 30 - 45°
- Frequent suctioning
- H$_2$ blockers and antacids to ↓ gastric acidity
- NG tube
- Bronchoscopy may be needed to remove as much particulate material as possible

(3) Pneumonia in AIDS

Pneumocystis carinii pneumonia (PCP)
- Most common opportunistic pneumonia in patients with AIDS (~ 80%). It is a fungus (not protozoa) that only causes disease in immunocompromised hosts
- ↑ Risk for this pneumonia when CD4 lymphocytes ↓ to < 200/mm^3
- Clinical presentation: gradual onset of fever, cough, dyspnea, diffuse infiltrates on CXR

Diagnosis
- Sputum stain induced by inhalation of hypertonic saline usually makes definitive diagnosis of PCP
- BAL fluid should be obtained if induced sputum is either negative or unavailable

Treatment
- Trimethoprim-sulfamethoxazole (TMP-SMX) (Bactram, Septra)
  15 mg/kg/d x 3 weeks?
- Pentamidine (IV 3 - 4 mg/kg/d x 2 weeks) if TMP-SMX not tolerated
  May also be aerosolized for mild disease
- Clindamycin-primaquine or atovaquone as other alternatives
- Corticosteroids during 1st 3 days of antibiotic therapy (e.g. prednisone
  40 mg bid x 5d then taper)
- O$_2$ for hypoxemia

Other pathogens often causing pneumonia in AIDS patients include cytomegalovirus (CMV), TB, common bacteria and fungi (esp. cryptococci and coccidioides).

10.1.3 Fungal pneumonia

NOTE: Treatment guidelines for all fungal infections below are based on IDSA/ CID recommendations (2000); see references at end of chapter.

10.1.4 Aspergillosis

Epidemiology and etiology
- Cause: *Aspergillus fumigatus*, which is transmitted by inhalation. It is a ubiquitous saprophyte fungus found in soil and water. Characterized by 45° branching points
- Often occurs in debilitated and immunocompromised hosts
  Causes: aspergilloma, allergic bronchopulmonary aspergillosis (ABPA), or invasive aspergillosis

Clinical manifestations
Aspergilloma ('fungus-ball'):
- Grows in areas of pre-existing lung cavities (e.g. old TB, sarcoid)
- Chronic cough, hemoptysis, dyspnea
- CXR: 'crescent-shaped' cavity around fungus ball

ABPA:
- Found only in asthmatics (5 - 10%) if steroid dependent and cystic fibrosis (CF) patients
- Wheeze, fever, cough, expectoration of fungus-containing mucus plugs
- CXR: infiltrates

Invasive aspergillosis:
- Restricted to immunocompromised hosts, especially neutropenic, chronic illness, long-term antibiotics or corticosteroid use
- High mortality
- Cough, fever, tachypnea, purulent secretions, pleuritic chest pain, ± hemoptysis
- CT scan: 'halo-like' lesion (crescent formation)
- CXR: local or diffuse infiltrates ± pulmonary infarction

Diagnosis
Aspergilloma:
- Does not cause many laboratory abnormalities
- Usually, +ve *Aspergillus* precipitin antibodies (IgG)

ABPA:
- +ve skin test to *A. fumigatus*
- Atopy: ↑ IgE
- Eosinophilia
- Anti-aspergillus IgE and IgG

Invasive aspergillosis:
- Observation of branching septate hyphae in tissue biopsy
- Using Gomori methenamine silver stain or +ve culture from sputum/BAL fluid/
  needle biopsy

Treatment

Aspergilloma

Surgical resection
- Definitive therapy, but has high morbidity and mortality and should be reserved
  for high-risk patients (e.g. life-threatening hemoptysis)
- Surgical candidates should have adequate pulmonary function

Bronchial artery embolization
- Possibly useful as a temporary measure in patients with life-threatening
  hemoptysis
- Procedure where vessel(s) that supply bleeding site(s) are occluded

Additional therapy
- Radiation therapy
- Intracavitary or endobronchial instillation of antifungal agents
- Inhaled nebulized antifungal agents
- Systemic antifungal agents

ABPA

- **Corticosteroids** (prednisone ~ 0.5 mg/kg/d) for acute exacerbations
- **Itraconazole** (Sporanox) as a steroid-sparing agent

Invasive aspergillosis

Antifungal agents
- Amphotericin B 1 - 1.5 mg/kg/d IV
  (use lipid-based amphotericin B for renal impairment)
- Itraconazole PO is an alternative to amphotericin B for patients who can take oral
  medications
- Voriconazole IV (6 mg/kg q12 h infused over 2 hours for 2 doses); maintenance
  dose 4 mg/kg IV q12 h if over 2 hours; when able, switch to 200 mg PO q12 h

Adjunctive therapy may be useful in certain situations
- Surgical excision
- Combination chemotherapy
- ± Immunotherapy

10.1.5 Blastomycosis

Epidemiology and etiology

- *Blastomyces dermatitidis* is endemic in southeastern and upper-midwestern USA (Ohio and Mississippi River valleys). It favors decaying organic matter and high humidity
- Transmission: inhalation of aerosolized conidia fungus, which converts to yeast once in the lungs. May disseminate through blood and lymphatics
- Blastomycosis is usually self-limiting in healthy people. Widely disseminated disease is most common in immunocompromised hosts (especially AIDS) and the elderly

Clinical presentation

- Pulmonary infection may be **asymptomatic** in ~ 50% of cases
- **Symptomatic** disease: flu-like illness: fever, myalgia, headache and nonproductive cough resolving within few days
- Chronic illness: fever, chills, pleuritic chest pain, myalgia, productive cough, weight loss, night sweats, ± hemoptysis
- CXR: alveolar infiltrates in upper lobes; often nodular; cavities in $1/3$ of cases; mass lesions (15%) mimic lung cancer
- Extrapulmonary: in up to $2/3$ of patients with chronic blastomycosis; most frequently affected sites are:
  ○ Skin: most common extrapulmonary site involved (20 - 40%)
  ○ Bones/joints: 10 - 40%
  ○ Genitourinary system: 10 - 25% (prostatic involvement is common)
  ○ CNS: ~ 5% (40% in AIDS patients)

Diagnosis

- Definitive diagnosis requires growth of organism from specimen from involved sites
- Visualization of characteristic appearance of budding yeast supports diagnosis of blastomycosis
- Serologic tests are not helpful as they lack sensitivity and specificity
- Bronchoscopy, cerebrospinal fluid (CSF) or blood specimens +ve

Treatment (based on illness severity)		
Type	Preferred	Alternative
Pulmonary		
Life-threatening	**Amphotericin B:** 0.7 - 1 mg/kg/d [total dose: 1.5 - 2.5 g]	**Amphotericin B** then **Itraconazole** when patient stabilizes
Moderate	**Itraconazole:** 200 - 400 mg/d (≥ 6 months)	**Ketoconazole:** 400 - 800 mg/d (6 - 12 months) or **Fluconazole:** 400 - 800 mg/d
Disseminated (extrapulmonary)		
CNS	**Amphotericin B:** total dose ≥ 2 g	**Fluconazole:** 800 mg/d if unable to tolerate full course of Amphotericin B
Non-CNS	Life-threatening or moderate: same as pulmonary	
Special circumstances		
Pregnancy	Amphotericin B 1.5 - 2.5 g (never use azoles for these patients)	
Pediatrics	Amphotericin B: total dose ≥ 30 mg/d or Itraconazole 5 - 7 mg/kg/d	

10.1.6 Coccidioidomycosis

Epidemiology and etiology

- Infection caused by *Coccidioides immitis*, which is a soil-inhabiting fungus that is endemic in Arizona, S. California, W. Texas, New Mexico, Nevada, Central America (N. Mexico, Guatemala, Nicaragua, Honduras) and dry regions of S. America (Argentina, Venezuela, Paraguay)
- Coccidioidomycosis is also known as Joaquin Valley fever

- Route of transmission: inhalation of arthrospores (diameter 2 - 6 mm), which, once inhaled, develop into thick-walled spherules filled with endospores. When these spherules rupture, endospores are released, each of which may develop a new spherule ⇒ spread of infection

Clinical presentation

Primary coccidioidomycosis:

- Most infections are asymptomatic (~ 60%) and resolve spontaneously
- About 40% recover fully from clinically mild, influenza-like (flu) illness consisting of cough, fever, fatigue, chills, erythema nodosum, pleuritic chest pain ± friction rub and arthralgia
- CXR: patchy infiltrates, hilar or mediastinal adenopathy, pleural effusion in < 10% of cases

Chronic pulmonary coccidioidomycosis:

- Develops in ~ 5% of infected patients and is manifested by fever, weight loss, cough, chest pain, ± hemoptysis, chronic fibrocavitary pneumonia and nodules/cavities

Disseminated coccidioidomycosis:

- Occurs in < 1% of acutely infected patients
- Increased risk: immunosuppressed individuals (AIDS, high-dose corticosteroid therapy, lymphoma and organ transplant) and males from African and Filipino descent
- Extrapulmonary dissemination may frequently involve skin, skeletal system and meninges

Diagnosis

Diagnosis can be made from direct microscopic visualization of spherules in patient's sputum, tissue biopsies or CSF.

- **Sputum culture:** isolating and identifying organism/spherules in sputum establishes diagnosis. Organism usually grows in 3 - 5 days on fungal media. Do not rule out if culture is negative
- **Bronchoscopy:** can be used when noninvasive techniques do not yield diagnosis. This may be the case in patients with parenchymal infiltrates or cavitary lesions. Transthoracic needle biopsy may be useful if bronchoscopy is not helpful

- **Serologic tests:**
  - Precipitin test: IgM antibody is detectable in 90% of patients within 4 weeks after the onset of symptoms
  - Complement fixation test for IgG anticoccidioidal antibodies:
    titers ≥ 1:4 in serum = current or recent infection. Titers > 1:16 suggest severe infection and increased likelihood of extrapulmonary dissemination. With successful therapy, titers decrease
  - Antibody detection in CSF is valuable in diagnosing meningitis
- **Coccidioidin skin tests:** delayed hypersensitivity is detected by injecting 0.1 ml of coccidioidin intradermally and measuring induration of ≥ 5 mm in 1 - 2 days

Treatment

1		Primary respiratory infections (controversial therapy)
	A	**Uncomplicated**
		• Most patients do not need therapy; periodic reassessment of symptoms and CXR findings is all that is needed
		• Risk factors (e.g. HIV organ transplant or high doses of corticosteroids) or unusually severe infections warrant initiation of antifungal therapy
		• Indications of severity: weight loss > 10%, night sweats > 3 weeks, infiltrations in > ½ of 1 lung or parts of both lungs, persistent hilar adenopathy, complement-fixing antibody to *C. immitis* > 1:16, unable to work or symptoms > 2 months
		○ Therapy: azole antifungals at their recommended doses for 3 - 6 months
		• Diagnosis of primary infection during 3rd trimester of pregnancy, consider therapy
		○ Amphotericin B is the treatment of choice during pregnancy because fluconazole and probably other azole antifungals are teratogenic
	B	**Diffuse pneumonia**
		• Initially amphotericin B for several weeks. Can be discontinued or replaced with azole antifungals
		• Total length of therapy should be at least 1 year and for patients with severe immunodeficiency, azoles should be continued as secondary prophylaxis

2		**Pulmonary nodule, asymptomatic**

- If a solitary nodule is due to *C. immitis*, antifungal therapy or resection is unnecessary
- In the absence of immunosuppression, antifungal therapy is not recommended if the lesion is completely resected

3		**Pulmonary cavity**
	A	**Asymptomatic**

- Many cavities due to *C. immitis* are benign and do not require therapy; with the passage of time, some cavities disappear, obviating the need for intervention
- Eventual resection from 1 to several years after cavity identification may be needed in order to avoid future complications, especially if the cavity is still detectable after 2 years, if it enlarges or if it is adjacent to the pleura

	B	**Symptomatic**

- Complications of coccidioidal cavities include: local discomfort, superinfections with other fungi, ± hemoptysis. This situation may benefit from **azole antifungals**
- If the surgical risk is not high, **resection** of localized cavities will probably resolve the problem

	C	**Ruptured**

- Pyopneumothorax: infrequent, but well-recognized complication occurring when coccidioidal cavity ruptures into pleural space
  - **Surgical closure** by lobectomy is the preferred management in young healthy patients
  - **Antifungal therapy** is recommended for coverage
- For patients for whom diagnosis is delayed ≥ 1 week or in whom there are coexisting diseases:
  - **Amphotericin B** or azole antifungal course before surgery or
  - Chest drainage without surgery

4	**Chronic fibrocavitary pneumonia**
	• **Fluconazole** 400 mg/d (if the patient improves, therapy should be continued for ≥ 1 year) • If therapy is unsatisfactory: switch to alternative azole antifungal, ↑ fluconazole dose or switch to amphotericin B • **Surgical resection:** may be useful for refractory well-localized lesions or where significant hemoptysis has occurred
5	**Disseminated infection, extrapulmonary**
A	**Nonmeningeal**
	• Ketoconazole, itraconazole or fluconazole 400 mg/d (alternative: amphotericin B, especially if lesions worsen) • **Surgical debridement** is occasionally important adjunctive measure
B	**Meningitis**

	• **Fluconazole** 400 - 800 mg/d (for life) or **itraconazole** 400 - 600 mg/d as an alternative
	• Hydrocephalus requires shunt for decompression
	   ○ May develop regardless of therapy being used
	   ○ If unresponsive to fluconazole or itraconazole, **intrathecal amphotericin B** 0.01 - 1.5 mg ± continuation of azoles is recommended

10.1.7 Cryptococcosis

Epidemiology and etiology
- Often found in areas contaminated with avian (pigeon) droppings. About 10% of AIDS patients develop cryptococcal disease
- Cause: *Cryptococcus neoformans*, an encapsulated yeast which is transmitted by inhalation

Clinical presentations

- In most cases, it disseminates to the CNS, usually without pulmonary involvement. Disseminated cryptococcosis usually occurs in hosts with impaired immunity:
  - AIDS patients
  - Prolonged corticosteroid use
  - Organ transplantation
- Meningitis: most common extrapulmonary cryptococcosis (90%)
  - Fever
  - Headache
  - Mental status changes
  - Neck stiffness
- Most common non-CNS infections:
  - Lungs: fever, cough, dyspnea, pleuritic chest pain
  - Skin: cellulitis, erythematous papules or pustules
  - Lymph nodes: lymphadenitis

Diagnosis

- Blood and serum cryptococcal antigens +ve in > 90% meningitis cases
- CSF with CNS disease shows: ↓ glucose, ↑ protein and WBC $\geq 20,000/mm^3$
- India ink is used to identify organism in CSF

Treatment

1	Cryptococcal disease in HIV -ve Patients
A	Pulmonary disease

NOTE: *In immunocompetent hosts, careful observation may be all that is needed, as the disease usually resolves without therapy.*

(a) Mild-to-moderate symptoms:
- **Fluconazole** 200 - 400 mg/d x 6 - 12 months or **itraconazole** 200 - 400 mg/d x 6 - 12 months if fluconazole not tolerated
- **Amphotericin B** 0.7 - 1 mg/kg/d (total dose 1000 - 2000 mg) x 6 - 10 weeks if oral azoles not tolerated or if disease is severe/ progressing

(b) Severe symptoms and immunocompromised hosts: treat as CNS disease (below)

	B	CNS disease (usually meningitis)
		• **Amphotericin B** (0.7 - 1 mg/kg/d) + **flucytosine** (100 mg/kg/d) x 2 weeks 'induction', then **fluconazole** (400 mg/d) x minimum 10 week 'consolidation'
		• **Alternative:** Amphotericin B + flucytosine or amphotericin B alone x 6 - 10 weeks (same doses as above)
		○ need lumbar puncture after 2 weeks of therapy to assess CSF sterility; if culture +ve may need longer course therapy (fluconazole 200 mg/d x 6 - 12 months is an option)
		○ Lipid form amphotericin B (AmBisome) 3 - 6 mg/kg/d should be used in renal disease
		○ **Surgery** may be needed for large (> 3 cm) accessible CNS lesions
		○ Intrathecal amphotericin B may be needed as last resort when systemic antifungals have failed
2		Cryptococcal disease in HIV +ve patients
	A	Pulmonary disease
		• **Fluconazole** 200 - 400 mg/d for life or itraconazole 200 - 400 mg/d as an alternative
		• **Fluconazole** 400 mg/d + **flucytosine** 100 - 150 mg/kg/d x 10 weeks
	B	CNS disease (usually meningitis)
		• Induction/consolidation: **Amphotericin B** (0.7 - 1 mg/kg/d) + **flucytosine** (100 mg/kg/d) x 2 weeks, then **fluconazole** (400 mg/d) x minimum 10 weeks, followed by **fluconazole** for life
		• **Alternative:** **Amphotericin B** (0.7 - 1 mg/kg/d) + flucytosine (100 mg/kg/d) x 6 - 10 weeks then fluconazole (400 mg/d) maintenance therapy
		• **Lipid** form **Amphotericin B** (AmBisome) 3 - 6 mg/kg/d x 6 - 10 week for renal disease
		• Maintenance: **fluconazole** (200 - 400 mg/qd PO) for life or **itraconazole** (200 mg bid PO) for life if intolerant to fluconazole

10.1.8 Histoplasmosis

Epidemiology and etiology
- Endemic in Ohio and Mississippi River valleys
  - Usually self-limiting disease with few or no symptoms
  - Symptomatic patients are usually immunocompromised (e.g. AIDS: very common) or are exposed to high amount
- Cause: *Histoplasma capsulatum*, a dimorphic fungus that remains in mycelial form and grows as yeast at body temperature. May spread to other organs via lymphatics
  - **Source:** soil contaminated with bird and bat droppings, which enhance growth of organism
- Transmission: Inhalation; air currents can carry spores for many km

Clinical presentation
Depends on severity of illness (host immunity and size of inoculum)

Acute pulmonary histoplasmosis:
  - ~ 90% of cases are asymptomatic
  - Common: fever, malaise, headache, cough, weight loss, pleuritic chest pain
  - Possibly: joint pain and skin lesions (< 5%), pleural effusion (<10%), enlarged hilar and mediastinal lymph nodes (5 - 10%), ± hemoptysis
  - CXR: infiltrates, hilar/mediastinal lymphadenopathy and rarely pleural effusion

Chronic pulmonary histoplasmosis:
  - Occurs mostly in patients with underlying pulmonary disease
  - Signs and symptoms: cough, weight loss, fever, malaise, ± crackles and wheeze
  - ~ 90% develop cavities that may enlarge and ⇒ necrosis
  - If untreated, may ⇒ progressive pulmonary fibrosis
  - May resemble post-primary TB

Progressive disseminated histoplasmosis:
  - Occurs mainly in immunocompromised and the very elderly
  - ~ 50% have mouth and gum pain due to mucosal ulcers
  - CNS involvement (5 - 20%) may produce: headache, confusion, altered LOC, neck stiffness and seizures
  - Acute form may produce: fever, worsening cough, weight loss, dyspnea and malaise

Diagnosis

- Sputum culture +ve in ~ 15% of cases with acute pulmonary histoplasmosis
- Blood culture +ve in 50 - 90% in acute progressive disseminated histoplasmosis
- Complement-fixing antibodies
  - Titers +ve when > 1:8
  - > 1:32 suggests active histoplasmosis infection
- Demonstration of organism on culture from involved sites to make definitive diagnosis:
  - Wright-Giemsa stain
  - Gomori's silver stain +ve in 50 - 70% of cases
- Cultures (lumbar puncture) +ve in 30 - 60% of histoplasma meningitis cases

Treatment		
Acute pulmonary histoplasmosis	**Chronic pulmonary histoplasmosis**	**Disseminated histoplasmosis**
Moderate manifestations: 1) None, usually benign 2) Itraconazole (200 mg once/d x 6 - 12 weeks) if symptoms > 1 month	Moderate manifestations: 1) **Itraconazole** (200 mg 1 - 2 x /d for 12 - 24 months)	Non-AIDS (moderate manifestations): 1) **Amphotericin B** then 2) **Itraconazole** for 6 - 18 months
Severe manifestations: 1) **Amphotericin B** (0.7 mg/kg/d) 2) **Prednisone** (60 mg/d x 2 weeks) 3) Itraconazole (200 mg 1 - 2 x /d for 12 weeks) after discharge	Severe manifestations: 1) **Amphotericin B** (50 mg or 0.7 mg/kg/d)	Non-AIDS (severe manifestations): 1) **Itraconazole** for 6 - 18 months AIDS (moderate manifest.): 1) **Itraconazole** for life AIDS (severe manifest.): 1) **Amphotericin B** then 2) **Itraconazole** for life

NOTE: *Fluconazole 200 - 400 mg/d can be used if patient cannot receive itraconazole; itraconazole is not recommended for meningitis.*

10.2   Lung Abscess

Definition
Localized cavity (a few mm or few cm) in lung parenchyma filled with pus

Causes
- Usually follows aspiration (absent gag reflex, sedation, loss of consciousness); therefore, normal mouth flora is often involved: *Klebsiella, Staphylococcus, Streptococcus, Pseudomonas*, etc.
- Also: inadequately treated pneumonia and bronchial obstruction (tumor, foreign body) may cause lung abscess

Signs and symptoms
- Malaise, weight loss, cough ± large amount of fetid purulent sputum, fever, pleuritic chest pain, ↑ WBC
- CXR: air-fluid filled cavity in lung parenchyma
- On affected side: ↓ ± bronchial breath sounds, dullness to percussion and crackles
- Should differentiate from TB cavity

Diagnosis
- Gram's stain
- Bronchoscopy with BAL or brush biopsy
- Percutaneous needle lung aspiration

Treatment
- Antibiotics: clindamycin [Cleocin]: 450 - 900 mg IV q8 h until afebrile x 1 week, then PO x 1 - 2 months. Most patients respond to antibiotics
- Postural drainage
- Oxygen for any hypoxemia

10.3   Tuberculosis (TB)

Etiology
- Infectious disease caused by *Mycobacterium tuberculosis* (aerobe), which is spread by inhaling airborne droplets (talking, coughing, sneezing)
- Usually involves upper lungs (apex) due to high V/Q ratio (higher O_2)
- *Mycobacterium* is ingested by macrophages in alveoli and transported to lymph nodes, where the spread may be contained or *Mycobacterium* may disseminate via bloodstream

Epidemiology

- $1/3$ of the world's population is infected, but do not have the disease
- TB accounts for ~ 7% (3 million) of all deaths worldwide
- 15 - 20 million people have active disease, mostly in developing world: SE Asia, Africa, Latin America and Middle East
- In the USA: high incidence for TB occurs among the following:
  - African-Americans (33%)
  - Immigrants (35%)
  - Hispanics (20%)
  - Asians and Pacific islanders (15%)
  - Alcoholics, homeless and drug-dependent people
  - Nursing home residents
  - Debilitating conditions: TB is 200 times more likely to occur in HIV +ve people than in those without HIV infection

Clinical manifestations

- General: weakness, malaise, anorexia, night sweats, fever and leukocytosis
- Pulmonary disease: chronic cough, hemoptysis, dyspnea, swollen lymph nodes (palpation), crackles over affected area, dullness and ↓ breath sounds over involved area and chest pain

Diagnosis

- CXR = consolidation, cavities in apical regions, lymph node calcification
- Sputum positive for acid-fast bacilli (Ziehl-Nielsen) test
- Purified protein derivative (PPD) skin test
  Consider positive when:
  - > 5 mm induration with major risk factors: HIV infection, CXR suggests TB, recent contact with infectious host
  - > 10 mm induration with: IV drug user, immigrant from high-prevalence country, high-risk group (e.g. Black, Hispanic, native American) and resident of long-term facility
  - > 15 mm induration with any

Treatment

- **Respiratory isolation:** to ↓ Mycobacterium transmission via aerosolized bacteria until 3 consecutive sputum AFB smears -ve
- **There are 4 recommended drug regimens** for treating TB patients caused by drug-susceptible organism. Each regimen has an initial phase of 2 months,

followed by several options for continuation phase of therapy for 4 or 7 months
(See table below)

- **Initial phase:** 4 drugs initially for 6-month regimen
  - 2-month initial phase of isoniazid (INH), rifampin (RIF), pyrazinamide (PZA) and ethambutol (EMB)
  - EMB may not be used when drug susceptibility test results are unknown
  - If PZA cannot be used in initial phase of treatment (e.g. gout, severe liver disease, ± pregnancy), INH, RIF and EMB are given for 2 months
- **Continuation phase:** given for either 4 or 7 months
  - 7 months is recommended for/when:
    - Cavitary pulmonary TB caused by drug-susceptible organism and sputum culture at end of initial phase is +ve
    - PZA not used in initial phase
    - INH and RIF used once/week and sputum culture at end of initial phase is +ve.

Recommended regimens	Initial phase (2 months)	Continuation phase (4 or 7 months)
Option 1	INH + RIF + PZA + EMB[2] daily x 8 weeks	INH + RIF daily or 2 x/week x 18 weeks (DOT) or INH + RPT[1] once/week x 18 weeks
Option 2	INH + RIF + PZA + EMB[2] daily x 2wks, then 2 x/week, then 2x/week x 6 weeks	INH + RIF 2 x/week x 8 weeks (DOT) or INH + RPT[1] once/week x 18 weeks
Option 3	INH + RIF + PZA + EMB[2] 3 x/week x 8 weeks	INH + RIF 3x/week x 18 weeks (DOT)
Option 4	INH + RIF + EMB[2] daily x 8 weeks	INH + RIF daily x 31 weeks or INH + RIF 2x/week x 31 weeks (DOT)

EMB = ethambutol; INH = isoniazid; PZA = pyrazinamide; RIF = rifampin; RPT = rifapentine; DOT = directly observed therapy (for continuation phase when given 2 - 3 x/week)

1. Used only for HIV -ve patient with -ve sputum smears after 2 months of therapy without cavitation on initial CXR.
2. If (when) drug susceptibility test results are known and organism is susceptible, discontinue EMB.

DOSES: first-line TB drugs for adults

Drug	Daily	Twice/week (DOT)	Three times/week (DOT)
INH	5 mg/kg (300 mg)	15 mg/kg (900 mg)	15 mg/kg (900 mg)
RIF	10 mg/kg (600 mg)	10 mg/kg (600 mg)	10 mg/kg (600 mg)
PZA	18 - 26 mg/kg (1 - 2 g)	36 - 53 mg/kg (2 - 4 g)	27 - 40 mg/kg (1.5 - 3 g)
EMB	14 - 21 mg/kg (0.8 - 1.6 g)	36 - 53 mg/kg (2 - 4 g)	22 - 36 mg/kg (1.2 - 2.4 g)
RPT	10 mg/kg (600 mg) once/week for continuation phase		

Source: ATS/CDC/IDSA statement: Am J Respir Crit Care Med 2003; 167: 603-662

Treatment of latent tuberculosis (prophylaxis)

Indications

- Active disease ruled out with -ve CXR or sputum AFB
- PPD conversion from -ve to +ve within 2 years
- Contacts with active TB
- Past TB with inadequate therapy, but no active disease present
- CXR evidence of nonprogressive TB, but no active disease

Preventive therapy

- **INH** 300 mg PO qid x 6 - 12 months (12 months if HIV +ve or CXR consistent with previous TB infection)
- Alternative (DOT): **RIF** (600 mg/d) + **PZA** (2 g/d) x 2 months if patient not unable to tolerate INH
- **Pyridoxine** 10 - 50 mg PO/d to ↓ risk for peripheral neuropathy associated with INH

Treatment algorithms for TB

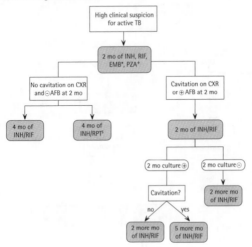

Fig. 23 Therapy algorithm for TB

EMB* : may discontinue when results of drug susceptibility indicate no drug resistance

PZA+ : may discontinue after 2 months (56 doses)

RPT^S : not to be used in HIV+ and TB or in extrapulmonary TB and therapy should be extended to 9 months if 2-month culture is +ve

Modified from/source: ATS/CDC/IDSA treatment of tuberculosis, Am J Respir Crit Care Med 2003; 167: 603–662.

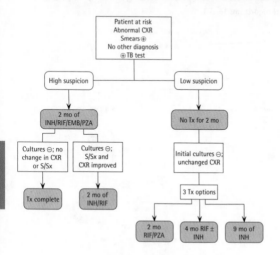

Fig. 24 Treatment algorithm for active, culture-negative TB and inactive TB

Modified from/source: ATS/CDC/IDSA treatment of tuberculosis, Am J Respir Crit Care Med 2003; 167: 603–662.

11. Interstitial Lung Diseases

Definition
- There are ≥ 150 types
- Injury of A-C membrane secondary to various known and unknown causes
  ⇒ regenerative process: inflammatory cells release mediators which increase
  fibroblasts and collagen deposition = ↑ A-C membrane thickness (fibrosis or
  scarring)

Etiology
- $2/3$ of ILDs not known

Known causes:
- Pneumoconiosis: asbestosis, berylliosis, silicosis, coal worker's pneumoconiosis
  (CWP)
- Toxic pneumonitis: chemicals, drugs, fumes, radiation therapy
- Respiratory bronchiolitis, malignant neoplasms, infections

Unknown causes:
- Sarcoidosis
- Pulmonary vasculitis (Wegener's granulomatosis)

Clinical Manifestations
- Progressive exertional dyspnea
- Tachypnea
- Crackles
- Dry cough
- CXR = varies widely - 'honeycomb'
- PFT: restrictive pattern (↓ lung volumes, ↓CL, ↓D_LCO, ↓/Normal FEV1/FVC)
- Hypoxemia secondary to exercise
- If advanced:
  ○ PH
  ○ Cor pulmonale

Diagnosis
Biopsy via fiberoptic bronchoscopy or bronchoalveolar lavage to sample cells from
distal airways

Treatment
- Corticosteroids may ↓ alveolar inflammation (fibrosis is irreversible)
- Avoid causative agent
- O_2
- Mechanical ventilation for RF
- Cytotoxic drugs

11.1 Idiopathic Pulmonary Fibrosis (IPF)

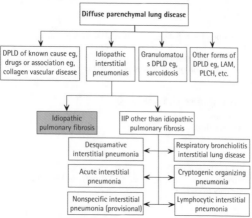

Fig. 25 Diffuse parenchymal lung diseases (DPLDs) consist of disorders of known causes (collagen vascular disease, environmental or drug related) as well as disorders of unknown cause. The latter include idiopathic interstitial pneumonias (IIPs), granulomatous lung disorders (eg, sarcoidosis), and other forms of interstitial lung disease (ILD) including lymphangioleiomyomatosis (LAM), pulmonary Langerhans'cell histiocytosis / histiocytosis X (PLCH), and eosinophilic pneumonia. The most important distinction among the idiopathic interstitial pneumonias is that between idiopathic pulmonary fibrosis and the other interstitial pneumonias (IPs), which include non-specific interstitial pneumonia (a provisional term), desquamative interstitial pneumonia, respiratory bronchiolitis-associated interstitial lung disease, acute interstitial pneumonia, cryptogenic organizing pneumonia, and lymphocytic interstitial pneumonia.

Description
End result of inflammation and repair (thickening of alveolar walls)

Incidence
Most common ILD: > 3 - 5/100,000

Etiology
Aspiration, infections, toxic gases, radiation, pneumonitis, autoimmune hepatitis or thyroid disease, TB, FIO_2 > 0.6 for > 48 hours etc.

Clinical features
- Progressive exertional dyspnea
- Dry (nonproductive) cough
- Malaise, weight loss
- Onset usually 40 - 70 years of age
- Fine inspiratory crackles on auscultation (especially at lung bases)
- Digital clubbing in > 65 - 70% of patients
- Cyanosis, tachypnea ± PH with loud pulmonary 2nd sound as disease advances

Diagnosis
- **CXR:** diffuse, bilateral, nodular or reticulonodular shadows mostly in lung bases. In advanced disease, honeycombing develops, with most lung areas being involved
- **PFT:** restrictive pattern: ↓ lung volumes (TLC, RV), ↓ lung compliance, ↓ D_LCO due to damage of pulmonary vascular bed and reduced lung volumes
- **ABG:** hypoxia, hypocarbia secondary to ↑ respiratory drive; hypercarbia in terminal stages. With exercise, there is widening of A - a gradient and ↑ hypoxia
- **Serum:** hypergammaglobulinemia, ↑ erythrocyte sedimentation rate (ESR), positive rheumatoid factor in ~ 30 - 35% of cases
- **BAL:** ↑ total cell count, ↑ neutrophils and ↑ eosinophils
- **CT scan:** may reveal abnormality before the CXR becomes abnormal. Reticular pattern is the most common CT appearance

Treatment
- **Immunosuppression:** corticosteroids (e.g. prednisone 1 - 2 mg/kg/d for 9 - 12 months) alone or combined with cyclophosphamide or azathioprine. About 25 - 35% of cases may respond to this treatment
- **Anti-inflammatory agents:** colchicines, plaquenil or chloroquine may also help
- **Supplemental O_2** for any hypoxemia

Prognosis
~ 50% die in 5 years. Range: 1 - 20 years

11.2   Pneumoconiosis: Occupational Lung Disorders

Parenchymal lung disease resulting from prolonged inhalation of work-related dusts

11.2.1   Asbestosis

Progressive diffuse interstitial fibrotic lung disease caused by chronic inhalation ($\geq$ 15 years) of asbestos (roofing material, heat insulation, demolition, ship building, etc.). Clinically resembles pulmonary fibrosis (nonproductive cough, crackles, clubbing, progressive dyspnea, PFTs: restrictive pattern with $\downarrow$ lung volumes and lung compliance, $\downarrow$ diffusing capacity [D_LCO]). Lung cancer or mesothelioma is a common complication. No treatment is available.

11.2.2   Berylliosis

Rare systemic poisoning by inhaled beryllium metal dust (electronics, nuclear weapons, high tensile alloys). Acute inhalation of beryllium dust may cause toxic or allergic pneumonitis. Symptoms are similar to sarcoidosis. Early treatment with corticosteroids may improve lung function. This disease is rare today as a result of strict control of beryllium in the industry.

11.2.3   Byssinosis

May be a form of extrinsic occupational asthma. Develops in workers who handle raw cotton and flax (linen). Unlike other pneumoconiosis diseases where inhaled dust causes alveolar reactions, inhaled cotton dust causes airway reactions. **Signs and symptoms:** acute bronchoconstriction with chest tightness, wheezing, dyspnea, and cough on exposure. This is possibly due to contaminating bacterial or fungal endotoxins. PFTs: obstructive pattern showing $\downarrow$ FEV$_1$, FEV/FVC ratio, FEF$_{25-75\%}$ and FVC, $\uparrow$ R$_{aw}$. There is no evidence of parenchymal involvement.
Long-term exposure may progress to irreversible airflow limitation similar to chronic bronchitis (productive cough and lung function decline).

11.2.4   Coal worker's pneumoconiosis (CWP)

['Black lung'] caused by deposition of large amounts of coal dust in the lungs. Clinical and radiographic features usually follow exposure by ~ 15 - 20 years. These patients often have chronic bronchitis. **Simple CWP** is characterized by small (< 4 mm) opacities found in the upper lobes of the lung. Simple CWP may lead to **progressive massive fibrosis (PMF):** characterized by fibrotic nodules > 1 - 2 cm. Patient shows breathlessness on exertion, irreversible airflow limitation, reduced lung volumes and ↓ D_LCO . Patient may also cough up black-tinged sputum.

11.2.5 Silicosis

Rare fibrotic lung disease caused by inhalation of silica dust. Occupations that may expose an individual to silica: sandblasting, brick making, stone drilling, quarrying, tunneling and hard-rock mining. Silicosis is usually seen in individuals who have > 15 years' exposure. **Simple silicosis** is characterized by small (< 9 mm) nodules scattered throughout the lungs and may cause no symptoms. **Advanced silicosis** is characterized by large nodules of fibrous tissue, usually found in upper lung zones, resulting in cough and severe dyspnea, especially on exercise. CXR may show 'egg-shell' calcification of hilar lymph nodes. Patients with silicosis are at ↑ risk for developing pulmonary tuberculosis.

11.3 Sarcoidosis

Description
Multiorgan disease with noncaseous granulomas of unknown etiology. It may affect any body part, but it most often involves lung, lymph nodes, liver, spleen, skin, eyes, joints and bones. Lungs are the most often involved organ in most patients (> 90%).

Incidence
In USA ~ 10 - 40 cases/100,000 (much higher in northern European countries such as Sweden); more common in blacks than whites

Etiology
Unclear; may be an inflammatory reaction caused by inhalation of bacteria, fungi, viruses or chemicals which occurs in people with genetic predisposition

Signs and symptoms
Thoracic sarcoidosis:
- About $\frac{1}{3}$ of patients have nonspecific features: fever, fatigue, anorexia, weight loss
- Dyspnea, dry cough and chest pain occur in 25 - 50%
- About 30% of patients have palpable peripheral lymph nodes (lymphadenopathy)
- About 50% of individuals with sarcoidosis are asymptomatic, but CXR is abnormal in > 90%. Radiographic classification of sarcoidosis:

Type 1: bilateral hilar lymphadenopathy
Type 2: hilar lymphadenopathy + parenchymal involvement

Type 3: parenchymal infiltration only

Type 4: endstage; advanced fibrosis (honeycomb lung, bullae, cysts, diffuse nodular pattern); < 3 - 5% of all cases

Extrathoracic involvement:
- Skin: (~ 25%) nodules, lupus pernio (macular lesions occurring on eyelids and spreading across the bridge of the nose)
- Eye: (~ 25%) glaucoma, lacrimal gland enlargement, corneal band opacities
- Heart: (~ 10%) most common cause of mortality in sarcoidosis patients (V-tachycardia, cardiomyopathy, complete heart block)
- Hepatic disease in ~ 25%
- Other: splenomegaly, CNS involvement (paralysis of cranial nerve VII), renal calculi, arthralgia, etc.

Diagnosis
- **Angiotensin–converting enzyme (ACE)** is often elevated, but this is not specific for sarcoidosis
- Endobronchial or transbronchial lung biopsy, bronchoalveolar lavage

Treatment
- Up to 50% of cases may resolve spontaneously within 3 years
- Corticosteroids **(prednisone)** are the traditional treatment
- Immunosuppressant 'steroid-sparing' agents such as **azathioprine**

11.4 Hypersensitivity Pneumonitis (HP)

Description
(aka extrinsic allergic alveolitis)

Diffuse inflammatory lung disease caused by repeated inhalation of dust composed of animal proteins, plant proteins or reactive inorganic compounds in sensitized individuals.

Causes
- Spore allergens of thermophilic actinomyces (*Thermoactinomyces vulgaris, Thermoactinomyces viridis,* Aspergillus species) in **Farmer's lung,** which is a disease of dairy farmers who handle contaminated hay during the winter months
- Avian proteins due to droppings or feathers in **Bird fancier's lung** or **Pigeon breeder's** disease

Clinical features
- **Acute:** fever, chills, nonproductive cough, chest tightness, dyspnea and malaise. These symptoms often resolve spontaneously within 12 hours to days
- **Chronic:** results from prolonged exposure to antigen which may lead to irreversible lung damage. Symptoms: gradually increasing dyspnea, malaise, weight loss and bibasilar crackles $\pm$ clubbing
- **CXR:** normal between attacks; nodular or reticulonodular pattern in chronic disease
- **CT scan:** 'ground glass' or honeycomb pattern in presence of fibrosis (chronic disease)
- **PFT:** may be normal between attacks; in chronic disease: restrictive pattern with $\downarrow D_LCO$, $\downarrow CL$, $\downarrow FVC$

Diagnosis
- Typical clinical course
- Positive precipitating IgG antibodies
- Bronchoscopy with transbronchial biopsy, bronchoalveolar lavage (lymphocytosis)

Treatment
- Avoid exposure to allergens; if unable, wear a fine mesh face mask
- Corticosteroids (prednisone): 0.5 mg/kg/d PO or 40 mg PO/day then taper

11.5 Lung Diseases Caused by Nonpulmonary Disorders

11.5.1 Wegener's Granulomatosis (WG)

Definition
Rare form of systemic vasculitis characterized by necrotizing granulomas and vasculitis of the upper and lower respiratory tracts. It is a multisystem disease consisting of the classic 'ELK' triad of:
1) **E**ars, nose, throat (upper respiratory tract)
2) **L**ungs (ILD)
3) **K**idney (glomerulonephritis)

Other organs that may be involved include: joints, eye, skin, heart, central and peripheral nervous system, GI tract and liver.

According to:
Am Coll Rheumatol (Leavitt RY et al: Arthritis Rheum 1990; 33: 1101-1107), presence of ≥ 2 of the following 4 criteria in patients with vasculitis classifies them as having WG:

1) Nasal/oral inflammation
2) Abnormal CXR (infiltrates, nodules, cavities)
3) Abnormal urinary sedimentation (hematuria)
4) Granulomatous inflammation on biopsy

Etiology
Unknown (autoimmune?)

Clinical features
- **ENT** (ear, nose, throat)
  - Rhinitis, sinusitis
  - Purulent and bloody nasal discharge ⇒ nasal obstruction
  - Nasal mucosal drying/crusting/ulceration
  - Septal perforation
  - Saddle nose deformity due to cartilage destruction
  - Also: otitis media, hearing loss, ear pain
- **Lungs**
  - Cough
  - Dyspnea
  - Hemoptysis
  - CXR: multiple nodules, diffuse alveolar pattern
- **Kidney**
  - Glomerulonephritis
  - Renal insufficiency
- **Eyes**
  - Conjunctivitis
  - Uveitis
  - Proptosis
- **Skin**
  - Necrotizing skin lesions
  - Purpuric rash
- **Joints**
  - Arthritis (usually large joints)
  - Myalgias; arthralgias

- **Central and peripheral nervous system**
  - Mononeuritis multiplex
  - Cranial nerve involvement/paralysis

Diagnosis
- **CXR:** nodules (1 - 9 cm in size), cavitated lesions, diffuse hazy opacities, ± pleural effusion
- **Laboratory investigations:**
  - Complete blood count: leukocytosis, anemia, marked ↑ ESR
  - Increased antineutrophilic cytoplasmic antibodies (ANCA):
    - ↑ cytoplasmic-ANCA (c-ANCA) in ~ 80 - 90% in WG patients
    - ↑ perinuclear-ANCA (p-ANCA) in ~ 10 - 20%
  - Urinalysis: ± hematuria, RBC casts and/or proteinuria
  - + Rheumatoid factor, ↑ C-reactive protein
- Biopsies of organs/tissues involved confirms diagnosis (lung is the most reliable source of tissue diagnosis). May sample lesions in the nasopharynx, if present

Treatment
- Corticosteroids and cytotoxic therapy:
  - **Prednisone** 1 - 1.5 mg/kg/d PO (~ 60 - 80 mg/d) **+ cyclophosphamide** 2 mg/kg/d PO
  - Taper prednisone over 1 - 3 month period once the disease is under control but continue cyclophosphamide for at least 6 - 12 months then taper dose in 25 mg increments q 2 - 3 months
- **TMP-SMX** (trimethoprim-sulfamethoxazole) 160 mg/800 mg PO bid may be an alternative for limited WG (lesions limited to upper and/or lower respiratory tracts without vasculitis and nephritis)
- **Methotrexate** (controversial) 0.3 mg/kg/week PO/IM (15 - 20 mg/week average dose) may be used as an alternative to cyclophosphamide in patients who do not have immediately life-threatening disease (no pulmonary hemorrhage or fulminant renal failure)

Prognosis
- About 90% of patients respond to cyclophosphamide and prednisone and ~ 75% achieve complete remission (but 50% experience relapses)
- 5 - 8-year survival is ~ 80% with aggressive therapy; without treatment, 2-year survival is < 20%

11.5.2 Systemic lupus erythematosus (SLE)

Definition

Multisystem, autoimmune inflammatory disease that can affect almost all of the organ systems. Incidence: 1/2000 individuals, with marked female predominance (M: F, 10:1). Most patients are diagnosed between 15 – 65 years of age.

Pulmonary complications of SLE:
- Pleuritis and pleural effusion (up to 60%)
- Acute lupus pneumonitis
- ILD
- Respiratory muscle weakness

Etiology

Unknown

Clinical features

- **Constitutional symptoms:**
  - Fever
  - Weight loss
  - Fatigue
  - Lymphadenopathy
- **Skin manifestations:**
  - Malar 'butterfly' rash
  - Discoid lesions: often begin as erythematous papules with scaling, then progress to follicular plugging and scarring. If present in the scalp, may lead to permanent alopecia
  - Reynaud's phenomenon may occur in 20 – 30% of cases
  - Photosensitivity: due to exposure to sunlight
- **Renal involvement:**
  - Renal disease (nephritis, acute renal failure, chronic renal insufficiency)
  - Evidence of renal disease:
    - Proteinuria: excretion of protein > 0.5 g/24 h
    - Presence of casts: RBC, Hb, granular, tubular
    - Increased serum creatinine
- **Musculoskeletal manifestations:**
  - Arthritis and rheumatism
  - Tendinitis
  - Arthralgia, myalgia

- **Pulmonary manifestations:**
  - Pleuritis with pleuritic chest pain (50 - 80%) ± pleural effusion
  - Diffuse alveolar hemorrhage: rare, but life-threatening process
  - Acute lupus pneumonitis (< 50%)
  - Interstitial lung disease (pulmonary fibrosis) < 35%
  - Pulmonary hypertension
  - Pulmonary embolism
- **Gastrointestinal manifestations:**
  - Abdominal pain
  - Nausea, vomiting
  - Dyspepsia
- **Cardiac manifestations:**
  - Pericarditis (serositis)
  - Chest pain (precordial) and pericardial rub
- **Neuropsychiatric manifestations:**
  - Headache, psychosis, depression or dementia
  - Seizures
  - Convulsion
- **Hematologic manifestations:**
  - Anemia (30 - 60%)
  - Leukopenia < 4000 WBC/mm^3 (20 - 40%)
  - Lymphopenia < 1500/mm^3
  - Thrombocytopenia < 100,000 platelets/mm^3 (20%)

Diagnosis

Requires ≥ 4 of the possible 11 criteria as defined by Am Coll Rheumatology		
1	**Malar rash**	Erythema fixed or raised
2	**Discoid rash**	Raised erythematous patches with keratotic scaling/ follicular plugging
3	**Photosensitivity**	Skin rash due to reaction to sunlight
4	**Oral ulcers**	Usually painless to touch
5	**Arthritis**	Nonerosive in ≥ 2 peripheral joints; tenderness, swelling, effusion
6	**Serositis**	**Pleuritis** (Hx of auscultated rub, pleural effusion) or **pericarditis** (EKG, auscultated rub or pericardial effusion)
7	**Renal disorders**	**Proteinuria** > 0.5 g/d; **casts** of any type

8	Neurologic disorders	**Seizures** or **psychosis** (without cause)
9	Hematologic disorders	Hemolytic anemia, leukopenia (< 4000/mm^3), lymphopenia (< 1500 mm^3) or thrombocytopenia (< 100,000 mm^3)
10	Immunologic disorders	Anti-double stranded DNA (dsDNA) antibody (50 - 70%), anti-Sm antibody (≤ 30%) antiphospholipid antibody based on IgG/IgM **or** +ve test for lupus anticoagulant **or** false +ve serologic syphilis test (25%) for > 6 months' duration
11	Antinuclear antibody (ANA)	At any time in absence of drug-induced lupus (+ve ANA ≥ 90%)

Hochberg MC: Updating the ACR revised criteria for the classification of SLE. Arthritis Rheum 1997; 40(9): 1725.

Treatment

There is no cure. Goal of therapy is to control acute, severe flares and to suppress symptoms to acceptable level. Treatment depends upon what organ(s) is involved:

Skin involvement, musculo-skeletal (arthritis, arthralgias)	• Non-steroidal anti-inflammatory drugs (NSAID) - any • Hydroxychloroquine (Plaquenil)200 mg PO qd/bid • ± Prednisone 1 mg/kg PO qid • ?Methotrexate (Rheumatrex) 7.5 - 15 mg qwk as steroid-sparing agent • Avoid sunlight; sunscreen (SPF 15)
Resistant disease (e.g. CNS, renal involvement, pleuritis)	• Prednisolone 1 mg/kg PO qid or methylprednisolone (Solumedrol) 1 - 2 mg/d IV • Cyclophosphamide 1 - 2 mg/kg/d • Azathioprine 1 - 3 mg/kg/qid as alternative

Prognosis

• 5-year survival is 85 - 90% and 10-year survival is 75 - 85%
• Most SLE patients die from infections, lupus nephritis and renal failure

12. Neuromuscular Disorders

12.1 Amyotrophic Lateral Sclerosis (ALS)

Definition (aka Lou Gehrig disease)

ALS is a progressive motor neuron disease with loss/degeneration of anterior horn cells of the spinal cord. There is also extensive loss of Betz's cells and other pyramidal cells from the postcentral cortex. Spinal motor neurons are also affected.

> NOTE: ALS does not affect eye movement, which distinguishes it from myasthenia gravis.

Etiology

- Cause is unknown, but about 5 - 10% of cases are familial (autosomal inheritance)
- Incidence is ~ 2 cases/100,000 in USA with M:F ratio of 2:1

Prognosis

There is no cure for ALS and it is usually fatal within 2 - 3 years of diagnosis; life can be prolonged with ventilatory support up to about 5 years post-diagnosis. Most patients die of frequent aspirations, pulmonary infections and respiratory failure.

Clinical manifestations/diagnosis

- Progressive weakness of distal extremities; in some cases there is an earlier involvement of bulbar muscles
- Difficulty in talking and swallowing
- Spasticity
- Diaphragm weakness ⇒ RF
- Diagnosis is clear if there is obvious deterioration in ≥ 3 areas:
  o **bulbar** (jaw, face, larynx, tongue)
  o **thoracic** (wasted back muscles and unable to sit up without support)
  o **lumbosacral** (signs of leg and foot weakness). If not clear, EMG ± nerve conduction tests are required to confirm denervation

Treatment

Since there is no cure, treatment is mainly supportive:

- Bronchial hygiene therapy
- Antispastic agents [baclofen, tizanidine]
- Theophylline? To improve diaphragm strength
- Riluzone, an antiglutamate for prolonging tracheostomy-free survival

- TT and mechanical ventilation to prolong life. The need for ventilatory support should be discussed with the patient and family early in the course of the disease to prevent rapid decline in lung function

12.2 Guillain – Barré syndrome (GBS)

Definition
Progressive ascending (lower limbs toward head) paralysis of unknown cause.
It is often preceded by viral infections, followed, days or weeks later, by motor polyneuropathy. In severe cases, paralysis of the diaphragm and ventilatory failure can develop.

Etiology
- ? autoimmune demyelinating disease secondary to viral infections (CMV, Epstein – Barr virus, influenza). Lymphocytes and macrophages appear to attack and demyelinate Schwann cell/myelin in the peripheral nerves. GBS is also associated with mycoplasma and surgery
- ~ 10% of GBS patients have history of preceding GI illness due to *Campylobacter jejuni*

Incidence
1 - 2/100,000

Clinical manifestations
- Loss of deep tendon reflexes
- Areflexia
- Ptosis (drooping eyelids)
- Diplopia (double vision)
- Dysphagia (difficulty swallowing) = increased risk for aspiration and pneumonia
- Dysphonia (slurred speech)
- Parasthesia of lower limbs

Common complications
Pneumonia, recurrent aspiration, cardiac arrhythmias and pulmonary thromboembolic disease

Diagnosis
- Spinal tap: ↑ protein in spinal fluid without increase in number of leukocytes
- Progressive ↓ in V_C and MIP
- Slowed motor nerve conduction (electromyogram; EMG)

Treatment
- Closely monitor V_C and MIP (q4 - 8 h); intubate if V_C < 15 - 18 ml/kg and/or MIP < 30 cmH$_2$O
- Aggressive bronchial hygiene therapy to prevent and treat atelectasis
- Plasmapheresis may limit progression and accelerate recovery when given early
- IV immunoglobulin may also be beneficial if given early in the course of the disease
- Mechanical ventilation (preferably via TT) is needed for ~ 15 - 30% of cases
- DVT prophylaxis
- Corticosteroids are unproven and may be harmful

Prognosis
Most patients usually recover in weeks or months, but ~ 15% of patients have residual weakness. About 5% of patients never recover.

12.3 Myasthenia Gravis (MG)

Definition
MG is a descending paralytic autoimmune disease in which there is a reduction in the quantity of Ach receptors at the NM junction (NMJ). Antibodies block Ach or destroy receptor sites at the NMJ. It is characterized by fatigue and muscle weakness, with improvement following rest.

Etiology
- Circulating antibodies disrupt the chemical transmission of Ach across the NMJ by:
  - Blocking Ach from receptor sites of the muscle cell
  - Accelerating the breakdown of Ach
  - Destroying receptor sites
- It is not clear what causes the formation of antibodies, but the thymus gland is almost always abnormal: **thymoma** (thymus tumor) is found in ~ 15% of patients (autoantibodies may arise from the thymus) and ~ 75% of MG patients have thymus gland **hyperplasia**

Clinical manifestations
- Weakness commonly affects extraocular muscles (**ptosis, diplopia**), facial muscles (funny smile) and bulbar muscles (**dysphagia** = aspiration risk). As the disease becomes more generalized, weakness may develop in the limbs, which is usually more pronounced in the proximal parts of the extremities. Onset: usually gradual
- Symptoms may be exacerbated by exertion, infection, pregnancy, surgery or certain drugs such as NM blockers, aminoglycosides, propranolol, lidocaine, quinidine, corticosteroids and tetracycline

Diagnosis

- Symptoms + ↓ V_C (consider intubation when < 1 L) and ↓ MIP
- **Tensilon (edrophonium) test:** anticholinergic drug alleviates signs and symptoms of MG for ~ 10 min = confirmed diagnosis
- **EMG** shows declining action potential in certain patients after slow repetitive nerve stimulation
- **CXR or CT:** to rule out thymoma or thymic hyperplasia

Treatment

- **Thymectomy** for thymoma. Be vigilant for RF, because it occurs in > 50% of patients post-surgery. Serial V_C and MIP measurements should be performed to help detect the onset of RF
- **Anticholinesterases:** pyridostigmine, neostigmine; remember that tensilon is used only for diagnosis because it has a short duration of action
- **Steroids** (prednisone) to ↓ autoantibody formation. Azathioprine (Imuran) may be added as noncorticosteroid immunosuppressive drug
- **Plasmapheresis** may be beneficial in MG patients who are not responding to conventional treatment
- Mechanical ventilation when V_C < 15 ml/kg and MIP < 30 cmH$_2$O
- Bronchodilators to alleviate bronchospasm caused by cholinergic drugs

12.4   Botulism

Description

Rare paralytic disorder caused by toxin produced by *Clostridium botulinum* (found in soil). Often, the source of botulism is food poisoning, but it can also occur from wound infection with the organism. Botulinum toxin binds to Ca^{++} channels in presynaptic NMJ, which prevents Ach release.

Symptoms

- GI symptoms predominate first (nausea, dry mouth, vomiting, diarrhea, abdominal pain), followed by
- Blurred vision, diplopia and descending paralysis, including the respiratory muscles

Treatment

- Ventilatory support for respiratory failure
- Botulinum antitoxin
- ± Penicillin
- Surgical wound debridement
- Enemas and gastric lavage are other options for therapy

12.5 Tetanus

Description

Disease caused by *Clostridium tetani*, a Gram-positive bacillus (found in soil) that produces spores. These spores, when introduced into a wound, skin cuts or burns produce a toxin (tetanospasmin) which fixes itself to presynaptic terminals of spinal inhibitory interneurons and prevents the release of of the inhibitory neurotransmitters (glycine and γ-aminobutyric acid). This leads to rigidity.

Presentation

- Early in the disease, trismus (lockjaw) and facial rigidity producing expression called 'risus sardonicus'
- In severe cases, dysphagia, rigidity of the entire body and opisthotonos (arched body with hyperextended neck) and spasms which may cause respiratory arrest

Differential diagnosis

Meningitis, status epilepticus, strychnine poisoning

Treatment

- Antibiotics (e.g. penicillin)
- Debridement of the infected wound
- IV human tetanus immune globulin (it does not reverse symptoms already present, but it stops progression of symptoms)
- In severe tetanus, airway should be secured (preferably by tracheal tube, since jaw is usually too rigid for intubation and recovery takes weeks) and spasms should be controlled with sedatives (e.g. diazepam) and paralyzers

12.6 Poliomyelitis

Description

Currently a rare disease in the USA and developed world because of the development of the polio vaccine by Jonas Salk. This is a disease that is largely responsible for the development of mechanical ventilation (Polio epidemic in the 1950s in Scandinavia).

Etiology

Poliovirus infects motor neurons in the spinal cord and brainstem; it attacks anterior horn cells. This virus is present in water and sewage and it spreads from person to person via fecal-oral transmission.

Signs and symptoms

- 'Pre-paralytic' stage: fever (such as due to gastroenteritis), tachycardia, headache, vomiting, followed by acute paralysis
- If the brainstem is involved (bulbar poliomyelitis), hypoventilation, apnea and paralysis of muscles of swallowing and speech may occur (aspiration risk)
- It should be noted that only a minority of infected persons develop paralysis, which is asymmetrically distributed

Diagnosis

Virus isolated from sputum or feces

Treatment

- Supportive care for acute phase, including assisted ventilation (for ~ 25% of patients)
- Physical therapy to maintain joint mobility
- Measures to prevent decubitus ulcers

Prognosis

- Most patients recover some or all motor function
- < 10% of paralytic cases die, but the anterior horn cell loss is permanent
- Some patients undergo late deterioration in function decades after the acute illness (post-polio syndrome)

12.7 Duchenne's and Becker's Muscular Dystrophies

12.7.1 Duchenne's Muscular Dystrophy (DMD)

Description

Rapidly progressing and the most frequently encountered muscular dystrophy starts in childhood. It is an inherited X-linked recessive disorder, but ~ $\frac{1}{3}$ of cases are due to spontaneous mutations. DMD usually affects boys.

Signs and symptoms

Onset: 2 - 5 years. Seen in ~ 1/3300 male births

Characteristics

- First abnormalities are noted when the child starts ambulating: frequent falls, painless weakness, mostly in pelvic girdle and thighs
- Excessively used muscles (calves) overdevelop, while other, underused muscles are poorly developed

- Gowers' sign: in order to rise and stand erect, child pushes up with hands against knees
- As the child ages, weakness becomes more severe and by ~ 10 - 12 years of age, the boy is wheelchair bound
- **Joint contracture**s (especially ankles, but also knees and hips), **scoliosis** or kyphoscoliosis (due to wasting of spinal support muscles) and **recurrent pulmonary infections** (due to inadequate cough reflex) ensue

Treatment

Mainly supportive
- Surgical correction of scoliosis may help to partially correct restrictive ventilatory defect
- Splints on ankles
- Surgical contracture release of ankles ± knees and hip joints
- Proper nutrition: high-protein, low-calorie diet
- Assisted ventilation: prolongs life by a few years; usually when V_C < 1 L, assisted ventilation is required. May start with NIPPV initially
- Corticosteroids (prednisone) increase muscle strength and may prolong ability to walk by 2 - 3 years

Prognosis

Survival past age 20 - 25 years is rare. Most patients die of respiratory or cardiac failure.

12.7.2 Becker's Muscular Dystrophy (BMD)

Description

Another X-linked muscular dystrophy disorder, which is considered by some to be a much milder (slowly progressive) form of Duchenne's dystrophy

Presentation

- Patients can still walk by age 16 - 17 years, with some even walking by age 60 - 80 years
- There is hypertrophy of calf muscles
- Scoliosis, cardiac failure and joint contractures are less frequent

Survival

Up to 60 years, with a few up to 80 years

13. Pulmonary Vascular Disease

13.1 Pulmonary Edema

Definition

Excessive accumulation of fluid in alveoli

Etiology

- CHF (LVF), MI, valvular disease (e.g. mitral stenosis)
- ↑ Capillary hydrostatic pressure
- ↑ Capillary permeability or ↓ colloidal osmotic pressure

Clinical manifestations

- Dyspnea
- Orthopnea (dyspnea relieved by upright position)
- Pink frothy sputum (RBCs)
- Wheezing (cardiac asthma), basal crackles
- Tachycardia
- Diaphoresis
- Hypoxemia/hypocapnea
- ↑ PAWP (> 20 - 25 mmHg)
- CXR: ↑opacity ('bat-wing' or 'butterfly' pattern), ↑ vascular markings, cardiomegaly

Treatment

- **High FIO$_2$** (non-rebreather mask), pulse oximetry, obtain IV access
- **Diuretics** (furosemide) IV: 20 - 40 mg initially. May need to repeat up to 120 mg, depending on urine output
- **Intubation/mechanical ventilation** + PEEP if unable to oxygenate sufficiently with non-rebreather mask until edema resolves
- Semi- or sitting position and feet down to ↓ pulmonary blood volume
- **Vasodilators** (nitroglycerine) ~ 0.3 mg sublingually q5 min x 3 prn to reduce preload
- **Bronchodilators** (albuterol and ipratropium) to relieve bronchoconstriction
- **Inotropes** (dopamine or dobutamine) may be needed if hypotension prevails
- **Morphine** IV at 2 - 5 mg as needed to reduce anxiety

13.2 Pulmonary Embolism (PE)

Definition
Obstruction of the pulmonary artery or one of its branches by a blood clot, which is usually secondary to DVT arising from lower extremities. Blood clot moves through the right heart to the pulmonary circulation, where it lodges in one or more branches of the pulmonary artery.

Etiology
3 main factors:
- Blood stasis: immobility, CHF, surgery
- Vessel wall damage: surgery, trauma
- Hypercoagulation: ↑ blood viscosity
  - Polycythemia (COPD)
  - Sickle cell
  - Oral contraceptives
- High risk: surgery of hip or knee
- 10 - 15% of PE patients may develop pulmonary infarct (tissue death secondary to lack of O_2)

Incidence
- 500,000/year with 50,000 deaths/year (10%)

Clinical manifestations
- **Symptoms:**
  - Acute onset of dyspnea
  - Pleuritic chest pain
  - Cough
  - Syncope (fainting) in large PE
- **Signs:**
  - Anxiety
  - Tachypnea
  - Tachycardia
  - Accessory muscle use
  - ↑ Jugular venous pressure
  - ↓ BS on affected side, crackles/wheeze

Diagnosis

- **Arterial blood gases:**
  - ↓ PaO_2, ↓ $PaCO_2$ due to hyperventilation
  - ↑ A - a gradient
- **V/Q lung scan:**
  - Patient breathes radioactive gas (Xe 133) to measure ventilation and is injected IV with radioactive particles (Tc 99) to measure perfusion
  - Well ventilated area and ↓ or absent perfusion (dark area) suggests PE
- **CT scan** of thorax
- **D-dimer: increased levels**
  - A fibrin breakdown product is a sensitive but nonspecific marker of clot formation
- **Angiography**
  - Gold standard, but it is invasive; used to confirm PE with borderline V/Q scan
  - Radioactive dye is injected into PA via catheter while serial CXRs are taken
  - PE = dark area distal to embolus

Treatment

- **Anticoagulation:**
  - Heparin initially, then
  - Coumadin [warfarin] for long term: > 3 - 6 months
- **Thrombolytic agents:**
  - Streptokinase (Streptase)
  - Urokinase (Abbokinase)
  - Main indication: recent acute PE; may be effective up to 2 weeks after onset of symptoms
- **IVC filter** when anticoagulation is contraindicated secondary to bleeding problem and recurrent PE
- **O_2 (up to 100% initially)**

13.3 Pulmonary Hypertension

Definition

PH is a rare, progressive disease characterized by PAP > 25 mmHg at rest or > 30 mmHg during exercise

Etiology

Revised Clinical Classification of Pulmonary Hypertension (Venice 2003)

1. Pulmonary arterial hypertension (PAH)

1.1 Idiopathic (IPAH)
1.2 Familial (FPAH)
1.3 Associated with (APAH)
    1.3.1 Collagen vascular disease
    1.3.2 Congenital systemic-to-pulmonary shunts
    1.3.3 Portal hypertension
    1.3.4 HIV infection
    1.3.5 Drugs and toxins
    1.3.6 Others (thyroid disorders, glycogen storage disease, Gaucher disease, hereditary hemorrhagic telangiectasia, hemoglobinopathies, myeloproliferative disorders, spelnectomy)
1.4 Associated with significant venous or capillary involvement
    1.4.1 Pulmonary veno-occlusive disease (PVOD)
    1.4.2 Pulmonary capillary hemangiomatosis (PCH)
1.5 Persistant pulmonary hypertension of the newborn

2. Pulmonary hypertension associated with lung diseases and / or hypoxemia

2.1 Left-sides atrial or ventricular heart disease
2.2 Left-sided valvular heart disease

3. Pulmonary hypertension associated with lung diseases and / or hypoxemia

3.1 Chronic obstructive pulmonary disease
3.2 Interstitial lung disease
3.3 Sleep-disordered breathing
3.4 Alveolar hypoventilation disorders
3.5 Chronic exposure to high altitude
3.6 Development abnormalities

4.Pulmonary hypertension due to chronic thrombotic and /or embolic disease

4.1 Thromboembolic obstruction of proximal pulmonary arteries
4.2 Thromboembolic obstruction of distal pulmonary arteries
4.3 Non-thrombotic pulmonary embolism (tumor, parasites, foreign material)

5.Miscellaneous

Sarcoidosis, pulmonary Langerhans cell histiocytosis, lymphangiomatosis, compression of pulmonary vessels by adenopathy, tumor, fibrosis mediastinitis, or other process

From: Simonneau, G, Galie, N, Rubin, LJ, et al. Clinical classification of pulmonary hypertension. J Am Coll Cardiol 2004; 43:10.

Clinical manifestations

- Common exertional symptoms (reflect inability of heart to ↑ CO during activity): dyspnea, syncope, fatigue, chest pain or lightheadedness
- Cardiac:
  - Angina
  - ↑ P2 (loud pulmonic valve sound)
  - Tricuspid regurgitation
  - Jugular vein distension (JVD)
  - Peripheral edema (ankles)
  - S3 (right-sided 3rd heart sound)
- CXR: enlarged PA

Diagnosis

- **Echocardiography** (two-dimensional with Doppler flow studies) is the most useful test for diagnosing suspected PH
- Tests to evaluate for secondary causes of PH:
  - **EKG:** right-axis deviation with evidence of RV hypertrophy
  - **CXR:** enlarged hilar vessels (pulmonary arteries)
  - **V/Q scan:** normal in PPH; essential to exclude chronic pulmonary thromboembolic disease (will show segmental V/Q mismatching)
  - **PFT:** to establish obstruction vs restriction
  - **ABG:** to exclude hypoxemia and acidosis
- **Right heart catheterization** is a definitive test for diagnosis and determining the severity of the pressures in the pulmonary arteries. It will exclude congenital heart defects and is used to monitor and measure response to medications

Treatment

Anticoagulation

- PPH patient is at ↑ risk of chronic thromboembolism secondary to ↓ venous return and ↑ right-sided filling pressures
- **Warfarin (Coumadin):** 1 - 5 mg/d; target 1.5 - 2.5 international normalized ratio

Positive inotropic agents

- Controversial: for patient with RV failure associated with PPH
- **Digoxin (Lanoxin):** 0.125 - 0.5 mg/d PO

Vasodilators: to ↓ PVR

- Oxygen for hypoxemia
- Ca channel blockers (avoid verapamil):
  - **Nifedipine (Procardia):** 10 mg PO tid initially (not > 180 mg/d) or
  - **Diltiazem (Cardizem):** extended release: 120 - 240 mg PO qid, max 540 mg/d; sustained release: 60 - 120 mg PO bid, max 360 mg/d
- Prostacyclin
  - **Epoprostenol (Flolan):** 2 - 4 ng/kg/min IV initially, then ↑dose 1 - 2 ng/kg q2 - 4 weeks according to symptoms and tolerance
  - **Iloprost, inhaled** (prostacyclin analog), Europe: alternative to IV epoprostenol, but due to its short-term effects, need 6 - 9 inhalations (30 - 90 min) to achieve good results. Minimal systemic side effects
- **Treprostinil (Remodulin):** for PAH; 1.25 ng/kg/min SC continuous infusion initially; may ↑ to 2.5 ng/kg/min/week (not > 40 ng/kg/min)
- **Sildenafil (Viagra):** selective oral pulmunary vasodilator; useful for PH secondary to pulmonary fibrosis
- **NO, inhaled** (investigational): FDA approved for newborn persistent PH

Endothelial receptor antagonist

- **Bosentan (Tracleer):** for PAH and PPH: 65.5 mg PO bid x 4 week, then 125 mg bid

Lung transplant

- Considered for selected patients when all medical treatments have failed

Prognosis

- PPH: median survival age is 2 - 8 years from the time of diagnosis (highly variable)
- Mortality ~ 50% at 3 y for untreated PPH and ~ 65% at 5 years with epoprostenol

13.4   Cor Pulmonale

Description

Right ventricular hypertrophy (RHF) secondary to chronic PH, induced by chronic alveolar hypoxia due to lung disease - most commonly COPD. Chronic hypoxia leads to vasoconstriction of pulmonary capillaries, which results in PH, eventually leading to RV hypertrophy because it must work harder against ↑ PVR.

Clinical features

- Peripheral (ankle) edema
- Hepatomagely (hepatic engorgement): may lead to abdominal pain
- JVD
- Tricuspid regurgitation
- Polycythemia

Diagnosis

- CXR: signs of PH: cardiomegaly from enlarged RV and enlarged hilar vessels
- Echo-Doppler examination of the heart and pulmonary circulation
- Right heart catheterization: gold-standard for diagnosis of PH (cor pulmonale)

Treatment

- Goal: optimize treatment of underlying lung disease
- Oxygen therapy: reduces hypoxic pulmonary vasoconstriction (↓ PVR), which reduces PAP, leading to improved RV function
- Vasodilators (diltiazem or prostacyclin)
- ± Digitalis, diuretics may help control peripheral edema

14. Pleural Diseases

14.1 Pleural Effusion

Definition
Abnormal collection of fluid in pleural space

Etiology

Transudate:
- ↑ Transcapillary pressure
- ↓ Plasma oncotic pressure: CHF (most common), cirrhosis, hypoproteinemia
- Transudates are usually bilateral
- Transudates have:
  - LDH < 200 IU/dl
  - Pleural LDH/serum LDH < 0.6
  - Pleural protein/serum protein < 0.5

Exudate:
- ↑ Capillary permeability = protein-rich pleural fluid: pneumonia, TB, trauma, PE, surgery
- Exudates have:
  - Pleural fluid LDH > 200 IU/dl or
  - Pleural LDH/serum LDH > 0.6
  - Pleural protein/serum protein > 0.5
  - ± ↑ Protein (> 3 g) or ↑ WBC

Clinical manifestations
- Dyspnea
- Pleuritic chest pain
- Ipsilateral ↓ chest wall expansion
- Breath sounds: ↓/absent and/or bronchial sounds over affected area
- Dullness to percussion on affected side
- Trachea/mediastinum shift away from affected side
- **CXR:** obliterated costophrenic angle (> 200 - 300 ml detectable on PA film, smaller on lateral decubitus view)

Treatment
- Fluid drainage by chest tube or **thoracentesis** (see following table). Unlike PTX, chest tube is inserted at base (not apex) of pleural space, to drain liquid
- **Antibiotics (only when parapneumonic)**

- O_2
- **Pleurodesis** for recurrent cases: irritant agent (talc or tetracycline) is introduced in pleural space ⇒ inflammation and fusion of visceral and parietal pleuras

Categorizing risk for poor outcome in patients with parapneumonic effusions

Pleural space anatomy		Pleural fluid bacteriology		Pleural fluid chemistry[+]	Cat.	Risk of poor outcome	Drain-age
A_0 Minimal, free flowing (<10mm on lat decub film)[°]	AND	B_X Culture and Gram stain results unknown	AND	C_X pH unknown	1	Very low	No[++]
A_1 Small to moderate free flowing effusion (>10mm and <1/2 hemithorax)	AND	B_0 Neg culture and Gram stain[°°]	AND	C_0 pH ≥ 7.20	2	Low	No[**]
A_2 Large, free flowing (≥ 1/2 hemithorax)[+++], loculated effusion[***], or effusion with thickened pariental pleura [°°°]	OR	B_1 Pos culture or Gram stain	OR	C_1 pH < 7.20	3	Moderate	Yes
		B_2 Pus			4	High	Yes

[+] pH is the preferred pleural fluid chemistry test, and ph must be determined by a blood gas analyzer. If a blood gas analyzer is not available, pleural fluid glucose should be used (PO =glucose ≥ 60 mg/dL; P1 = glucose <60 mg/dL). The expert panel cautions that the clinical utility and decision thresholds for pH and glucose have not been well-established.

[°] Clinical experience indicates that effusions of this size do not require thoracentesis for evaluation, but will resolve.

[++] If thoracentesis were performed in a patient with AO category pleural anatomy and P1 or B1 status found, clinical experience suggests that the P1 or B1 findings might be false-positive. Repeat thoracentesis should be considered if effusion enlarges and/or clinical condition deteriorates.

[**] If clinical condition deteriorates, repeat thoracentesis and drainage should be considered.

[°°] Regardless of prior antibiotic use.

+++ Larger effusions are more resistant to effective drainage, possibly because the increased likelihood that large effusions will also be loculated.

*** Pleural loculations suggest a worse prognosis.

°°° Thickened parietal pleura on contrast-enhanced CT suggests presence of empyema.

Adapted from Colice, GL, Durtis, A, Deslauriers, J, et al, Chest 2000; 118:1158.

14.1.1 Hemothorax

Description
A collection of blood in the pleural cavity, which is usually of acute course. It is characterized by Hct value > 50% above that of serum.

Signs and symptoms
- Chest pain
- Dyspnea
- Tachycardia
- Asymmetrical chest movement
- Hypotension

Causes
- Frank bleed into pleural space
- Penetrating or blunt chest trauma: blood from laceration of the lung or intercostal blood vessels
- Hematologic disorders

Treatment
- Insertion of large-bore (38 - 40 Fr) chest tube placed in the midaxillary line between 5th and 6th intercostal space
- Chest tube is connected to chest drainage system and a continuous negative (suction) pressure of about - 20 cmH$_2$O is used

14.1.2 Chylothorax

Description
Chylothorax is characterized by passage of chyle (lymphatic fluid) from the thoracic duct into the pleural cavity. Damage to the thoracic duct (tear or trauma) ⇒ collection of chylous fluid in the pleural cavity.

Etiology

- Tumors: ≥ 50% of cases
  - Lymphomas are responsible for > 75% of malignancy-associated chylothoraxes
- Trauma: 2nd most common cause of chylothorax (≥ 25% of cases)
  - Surgery is the most common cause of traumatic (iatrogenic) chylothorax
  - Rare: penetrating trauma
- Rare causes:
  - Pulmonary lymphangioleiomyomatosis
  - Tuberous sclerosis
  - Congenital defect
  - Cirrhosis
  - Tuberculosis
- Etiology of chylothorax is unknown in ~ 15 - 25% of cases

Diagnosis

- Symptoms of chylothorax are usually minor until a large volume of chyle accumulates
- Signs and symptoms may include: dyspnea, tachypnea, decreased BS, shifting of dullness to percussion, while fever and chest pain are absent
- **Thoracentesis** to analyze pleural fluid:
  - Triglycerides > 110 mg/dl suggests chylothorax
  - Triglycerides < 50 mg/dl excludes chylothorax
  - In patients with triglyceride values between 50 - 110 mg/dl, a lipoprotein analysis of the pleural fluid is performed and if chylomicrons are present, the diagnosis of chylothorax is established
  - Fluid that is milky (white) and odorless suggests chylothorax, but not all chylous fluids are milky. Almost ½ are either bloody or turbid in appearance; therefore, evaluation of triglycerides is essential when the etiology is unknown
- **CXR:** nonspecific for chylothorax (check if effusion is bilateral and look for mediastinal shift)
- **CT scan:** if etiology is unknown to rule out malignancy

Treatment

- In many patients with traumatic chylothorax, there is no need for treatment, as the thoracic duct defect closes spontaneously
- For lymphoma or metastasizing tumor (patients who are not surgical candidates):
  - Irradiation of mediastinum or
  - Systemic chemotherapy

- For trauma:
  - **Pleural drainage** (thoracoscopy or repeated thoracentesis)
  - **Surgical ligation** of the thoracic duct if the lymph drainage has not stopped spontaneously within 5 - 7 days
  - **Pleurodesis** for some patients who are not surgical candidates
- Pleuroperitoneal shunt
- Total parenteral nutrition or a fat-restricted diet with triglycerides to decrease chyle formation

14.2   Pneumothorax (PTX)

Definition
Air accumulation in the pleural space as a result of air leak (extrapulmonary gas) from alveolar rupture = air leaks into interstitium and then pleura. In neonates, it often develops from blebs due to excessive pressure or volume, such as from PPV during resuscitation or mechanical ventilation.

Etiology
- **Spontaneous:** due to rupture of blebs, usually in thin tall young males with history of smoking
- **Traumatic:** iatrogenic (i.e. subclavian central line insertion, excessive PPV, thoracic surgery, transbronchial lung biopsy) or penetrating chest trauma (knife, bullet)
- **Tension PTX:** most serious: air enters on inspiration but cannot escape on expiration = ↑ PTX size with each breath ⇒ lung eventually collapses under increasing pressures

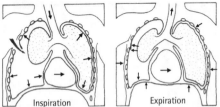

Fig. 26 Tension pneumothorax produced by chest wall wound. Air is able to enter through the wound on inspiration, but cannot escape on expiration. This leads to compression and collapse of the lung.

Inspiration   Expiration

Clinical manifestations
- Ipsilateral pleuritic chest pain
- Dyspnea
- ↓ or absent BS on affected side
- Hyperresonance to percussion
- ↓ Chest excursion on affected side
- With tension PTX: cardiac pulse shift away from affected area
- Cyanosis
- Hypoxemia
- Hypotension (late)
- Tracheal shift

Diagnosis
- **CXR:** no lung markings on affected side peripheral to edge of collapsed lung and depressed diaphragm, tracheal/mediastinal shift to unaffected side (tension PTX)
- **Transillumination** for newborns may help in diagnosis of suspected PTX (i.e. respiratory distress, ↓ ± absent respiratory sounds with tracheal shift) when rapid CXR is unavailable. It is used in darkened room; if the chest 'lights up', this suggests ↑ amount of air in the thorax. Unaffected lung is darker

Treatment
- **Small PTX:** usually asymptomatic and resolves spontaneously
- **Large PTX:** Requires immediate action of large-bore **needle aspiration** (14 - 16 gauge in adults) ± chest tube into 2nd or 3rd intercostal space anteriorly after local anesthesia. Syringe is partially filled with normal saline and the needle is inserted on the side of suspected PTX. Remove plunger to let trapped air bubble out through the syringe (saline acts as H_2O seal) until chest tube can be inserted, if needed

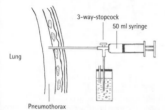

Fig. 27 Pneumothorax drainage through needle aspiration. Note that the needle is inserted immediately above the rib to avoid nerves and vessels which are located below the rib.

○ **Chest tube** is needed with moderate lung collapse (~ ½ way toward heart border), unresponsive to needle aspiration and complete lung collapse.
A 36 - 40 French chest tube is inserted into 5th intercostal space in mid-axillary line with 15 - 20 cmH$_2$O water seal suction. Drain should not be clamped and should be removed after the leak has sealed (~ 24 hours). If there is constant bubbling, there may be a leak around the drain tube, tube may be improperly placed or BP fistula may exist

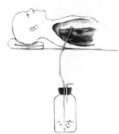

Fig. 28 Chest drainage system

• **Recurrent PTX** may need
○ Pleurectomy or **Pleurodesis:** injection of irritant such as talc or tetracycline into pleura to seal the pleurae together

14.3 Pulmonary Interstitial Emphysema (PIE)

Definition
Extrapulmonary gas within interstitial space. May cause compression of pulmonary vessels which ⇒ ↑ PVR and compression of lymphatic vessels = ↑ lung water

Etiology
• Often secondary to excessive PPV during mechanical ventilation in premature infants with RDS
• Predisposing factors: IRDS, MAS, lung immaturity, air trapping

Clinical manifestations
- Tachypnea
- Cyanosis
- Retractions in newborns
- CXR: 'bubbles' due to cyst formation ± air bronchograms

Treatment
- May clear spontaneously
- Lower ventilating pressures: ↑ RR, ↓ PIP (< 25 - 30 cmH$_2$O)
- If unilateral PIE, positioning the infant with affected side down may help
- Intermittent ↑ O$_2$ (100% oxygen for 10 - 15 min intervals) may help in absorption of extrapulmonary air
- High-frequency ventilation (HFV)?

15. Sleep Apnea

Definitions

- Apnea: cessation of airflow for ≥ 10 s
- Hypopnea: $\downarrow$ airflow by < 50% and O_2 desaturation
- Apneic index (AI): No. of apneic episodes/sleep hour
- Apnea hypopnea index (AHI): No. of episodes of apnea and hypopnea/hour
  - AHI > 10 is abnormal
  - AHI is also called respiratory disturbance index (RDI)
- Sleep apnea: > 6 apneic episodes/hour during sleep

Types of sleep apnea

1	Obstructive sleep apnea (OSA): 85 -90%	Cessation of airflow for ≥ 10 s with respiratory effort. Due to upper airway obstruction at pharynx
2	Central sleep apnea (CSA): 1 0 - 15%	Cessation of airflow for ≥ 10 s without respiratory effort. Due to impairment of respiratory center
3	Mixed apnea	Combination of OSA and CSA

15.1 Obstructive Sleep Apnea (OSA)

OSA is characterized by repetitive upper airway obstruction (lack of airflow despite respiratory effort) during sleep, often resulting in arousals and O_2 desaturations/hypoxemia.

Prevalence in the US: males (4%) > females (2%)

Etiology

- Obesity: $^2/_3$ of patients
  - Body mass index (BMI) > 28 kg/m^2 = $\uparrow\uparrow$ likelihood of OSA than in nonobese individuals
  - BMI = weight (kg) $\div$ height (m)
- Large tongue
- Short and/or thick neck: > 42 cm (16.5 in) circumference
- Micrognathia (small chin)
- Retrognathia (recessed chin)
- Deviated nasal septum
- Enlarged tonsils and/or adenoids (especially in children)

- Alcoholism, sedatives, hypnotics
- Hypothyroidism

Clinical features

- Excessive daytime somnolence (sleepiness)
  - Higher risk (7 x normal) of automobile accidents
  - Leads to ↓ work productivity, ↓ reaction time, ↑ chance of errors
  - Useful self-assessment of sleepiness (Epworth sleepiness scale) is shown below
- Loud snoring (due to partial obstruction)
- Witnessed apneas
- Mood and personality changes
- Poor concentration and cognitive impairment
- Impotence
- Headaches (especially morning)
- Obese (not always) $\frac{2}{3}$ of patients
- Systemic hypertension in ~ 50% patients
- Short, thick neck: > 42 cm
- Upper airway abnormalities:
  - Craniofacial malformations (e.g. macroglossia, micrognathia, retrognathia, large uvula)
  - Hypertrophy of tonsils and/or adenoids (common cause in children)
- Possibly PH, cyanosis and/or erythrocytosis in severe cases, but this is likely to be due to chronic hypoxemia

Epworth Sleepiness Scale

How likely are you to doze off or fall asleep in the following situations, in contrast to just being tired? Choose the most appropriate number for each situation below.
0 = Would NEVER doze
1 = SLIGHT chance of dozing
2 = MODERATE chance of dozing
3 = HIGH risk of dozing

Situation	Chance of Dozing			
Sitting and reading	0	1	2	3
Watching TV				
Sitting, inactive in public place				
Lying down to rest				
Sitting and talking to someone				

Sitting quietly after lunch without alcohol		
In a car, while stopped for few minutes in traffic		
In a car driving		
	SCORE:	

Interpreting total score:
< 8 = normal sleep function
8 - 10 = mild sleepiness
11 - 15 = moderate sleepiness
16 - 20 = severe sleepiness
21 - 24 = excessive sleepiness

Diagnosis

OSA may be diagnosed on the basis of clinical features, overnight pulse oximetry and/or video recording, but definitive diagnosis requires overnight polysomnography.

- **Polysomnography (PSG):** all night recording of several physiological signals to determine if the airway occlusion occurs during sleep and the extent to which it disturbs sleep and cardiopulmonary function. Variables to be monitored include:

Electrooculogram (EOG)	To record sleep stages
EMG	To record muscle activity (chin)
Airflow (nasal/oral)	Detected by thermistor
Respiratory effort (thoracic/abdominal)	Measured by magnetometers or impedance plethysmography
Pulse oximetry (SpO_2)	To detect desaturations
EKG	To detect HR and evaluate effects of apnea
Electroencephalogram (EEG)	To record sleep stages

OSA is usually diagnosed when patient has AHI > 5/hour and O_2 desaturation of $\geq 4\%$

OSA Severity	AHI	$SpO_2\%$
Normal	< 5	> 93
Mild	5 - 15	> 85
Moderate	15 - 30	65 - 84
Severe	> 30	< 65

• Split-night PSG study:
Initial part (e.g. first 3 hours of sleep) is used for diagnosis and the remaining part of sleep is used for constant positive airway pressure (CPAP) titration.
May be considered when AHI 20 - 40.

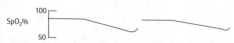

Fig. 29 Obstructive sleep apnea is characterized by cessation of airflow with respiratory effort (rib cage and abdomen movement) and O_2 desaturation. Central sleep apnea is characterized by the absence of airflow without respiratory effort and O_2 desaturation.

Treatment

Behavioral interventions

- Weight loss for overweight patients
- Avoid: alcohol, sedatives, supine position, sleep deprivation and smoking

Medical interventions

- **Nasal CPAP** during sleep ($\pm$ O_2): preferred method
  - Very effective in most cases, but ~ ½ of patients are noncompliant or not using it regularly
  - Pressure is titrated for effectiveness (e.g. 8 - 15 cmH$_2$O)
  - Side effects include: claustrophobia, nasal dryness, skin irritation and system leaks
  - Bilevel PAP (BiPAP) may be preferred over CPAP by some patients who complain about exhaling against elevated pressure during CPAP

- **Oral appliances:** for mild-moderate cases
  - Mandibular advancement splints
  - Dental splints
  - Tongue retainers

- **Pharmacotherapy:** may be effective in limited number of patients
  - Protriptyline 10 - 20 mg PO qhs to ↓ REM sleep
  - Theophylline
  - Progesterone may stimulate respiratory drive
  - Acetazolamide to enhance respiratory drive
  - O_2 therapy should be used with caution in patients that retain CO_2

Surgical interventions

- **Uvulopalatopharyngoplasty (UPPP)**
  - Excision of redundant tissue of soft palate, uvula and pharyngeal wall
  - May be effective in eliminating snoring, but often fails to control sleep apnea adequately
  - Success rate $\leq$ 50% (lower in obese patients)
  - **Laser-assisted uvuloplasty (LAUP)** may be successful for uncom-plicated snoring, but has not been shown to be efficient for OSA

- **Tracheostomy**
  - Bypasses obstructed areas and is 100% effective, but is unacceptable to many patients due to its disfigurement and lack of social acceptability
  - It is a last resort for severe OSA when CPAP is refused, not tolerated or is ineffective
- The following may help in selected patients:
  - Correction of deviated septum and excision of nasal polyps
  - Tonsillectomy: removing obstructing tonsils and adenoids
  - Mandibular advancement for micrognathia
  - Elevation of hyoid bone
- **Radiofrequency tissue volume reduction** (somnoplasty)
  - Procedure with the same objective as UPPP. Electrodes are inserted into the soft palate and behind the tongue. Heat energy from needle electrodes causes tissue to heat up, coagulate and over time ↓ its volume
  - Usually require > 1 procedure to be effective

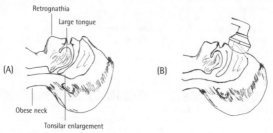

Fig. 30 Figure (A) shows factors predisposing to upper airway narrowing and OSA; Figure (B) demonstrates the effects of nasal CPAP: there is airway splinting and dilatation of obstructive pharyngeal tissues

15.2 Central Sleep Apnea (CSA)

Description

Unlike OSA, CSA is not a single disorder, but a group of disorders that manifest as central apneas during sleep. Much less common than OSA (may account for 10 - 15% of apnea patients).

Etiology

- Failure of respiratory center (medulla) to send signals: CVA, neurologic disease, brainstem disease
- Sleeping at high altitudes
- CHF

Clinical features

- Cheyne - Stokes breathing (usually due to CHF); it meets the definition of CSA, but the cause is probably different
- Ranges from daytime sleepiness, PH, cor pulmonale, polycythemia, to restless sleep

Diagnosis

High clinical suspicion and overnight polysomnography which demonstrates repeated episodes of apnea without respiratory effort

Treatment

- Nocturnal nasal CPAP is the treatment of choice
- Correct/improve CHF
- Respiratory stimulants (progesterone, acetazolamide) are not useful for conventional central apneas, but may be of benefit for CSA associated with high altitude
- Diaphragmatic pacer (controversial) for severe cases
- Low-flow O_2 (especially at high altitudes)

16. Lung Cancer

Etiology/Risk factors

Cigarette smoking:
- Accounts for 75 - 90% of all lung cancers
- Interplay between carcinogen exposure and host genetic susceptibility plays a role in some, because < 20% of smokers develop lung cancer
- Among ex-smokers, 10 years after smoking cessation, the risk of developing lung cancer is ↓ by 50%
- Long-term exposure to second-hand smoke ⇒↑ risk for developing lung cancer

Environmental/occupational exposures:
- Asbestos (sustained exposure)
- Radon, e.g. uranium miners or indoor radon that diffuses into homes built in areas containing high levels of uranium. ~ 14,000 deaths/year in the USA are attributed to radon exposure
- Also: aluminum byproducts, arsenic, chromium and nickel compounds (e.g. welding), bis-chloromethyl ether (painting; textile workers) and vinyl chloride

Comorbidities:
- Smokers with airflow obstruction, patients with IPF, history of TB and patients with head or neck carcinoma are at ↑ risk of lung cancer
- Also patients with previous lung cancer, ± patients with HIV

Clinical presentation
The presence of symptoms usually denotes advanced disease. A minority of patients (< 10%) come to attention because of asymptomatic CXR abnormality that was obtained for other reasons or as a part of screening evaluation.
- Most lung cancer symptoms are nonspecific
- The most common presenting symptoms are:
  - Cough ± hemoptysis; new cough or change in chronic cough is an important symptom in a smoker
  - Chest pain
  - Dyspnea
  - Constitutional symptoms
- Symptoms related to advanced spread of disease
  - Hoarseness (recurrent laryngeal nerve palsy) due to mediastinal invasion
  - Facial edema

- Superficial venous congestion: prominent venous pattern on patient's chest due to SVC obstruction caused by lung cancer
- Shoulder pain: direct neurovascular extension of apical Pancoast tumor
- Fixed wheezing or stridor suggests large airway obstruction
- Also: finger clubbing, fatigue, anorexia and weight loss
- CXR:
  - Solitary pulmonary nodule or mass
  - Hilar enlargement
  - Post-obstructive atelectasis, pneumonitis or hyperinflation
  - Mediastinal adenopathy
  - Bony destruction
  - Pleural effusion

Classification (Histology)

Small cell lung carcinoma (SCLC):

- Accounts for ~ 20% of all lung cancers; rapid growth
- Derived from neoplastically transformed neuroendocrine cells. Strongly associated with cigarette smoking
- Treatment primarily involves chemotherapy
- Usually central in origin (hilar region)
- Mortality/morbidity: 1 - 5% 5-year survival rate and median survival is 6 - 10 months

Nonsmall cell lung cancer (NSCLC):

- ~ 80% of all lung cancers
- Derived from transformed epithelial cells
- Surgical resection is a cornerstone of curative therapy
- NSCLC can be subdivided into:
  - **Adenocarcinoma (40%)**: usually presents as a peripheral lung nodule or mass; more common in nonsmokers; slow growing
  - **Squamous cell carcinoma (30%)**: strongly associated with tobacco use; usually central in location (e.g. large bronchi near hilar region); slow growth
  - **Large cell undifferentiated carcinoma (10%)**: may be found either in periphery or central regions of the lung; cavity formation is common
- Mortality/morbidity: 5-year survival ~ 14%

Staging of NSCLC

TNM (tumor, node, metastasis) descriptors

Primary tumor (T)	
TX	Cannot be assessed or +ve malignant cytology in sputum/bronchial washings, but not visualized by imaging or bronchoscopy
T0	No evidence of primary tumor
Tis	Carcinoma in situ
T1	≤ 3 cm surrounded by lung or visceral pleura, without bronchoscopic evidence of invasion proximal to lobar bronchus
T2	Tumor with any of the following features: • > 3 cm in widest diameter • Involves main bronchus, ≥ 2 cm distal to carina • Invades visceral pleura • Associated with atelectasis or obstructive pneumonitis that extends to hilum but does not invade entire lung
T3	Tumor of any size that invades any of the following: • Chest wall (including superior sulcus tumors), diaphragm, mediastinal pleura or parietal pericardium; OR • Tumor in main bronchus < 2 cm distal to carina, but without involving carina; OR • Associated atelectasis or obstructive pneumonitis of entire lung
T4	Tumor of any size that invades any of the following: • Mediastinum, heart, great vessels, trachea, esophagus, vertebral body, carina; OR • Malignant pleura or pericardial effusion; OR • Satellite tumor nodules within same lobe of lung

Regional lymph nodes (N)	
NX	Cannot be assessed
N0	No demonstrable metastasis
N1	Metastasis ipsilateral to peribronchial ± hilar lymph nodes and/or direct extension to intrapulmonary nodes

| N2 | Metastasis to ipsilateral mediastinal or subcarinal lymph nodes |
| N3 | Metastasis to contralateral mediastinal or hilar, contralateral or ipsilateral scalene or supraclavicular lymph nodes |

Distant metastasis (M)	
MX	Cannot be assessed
M0	None (unknown)
M1	Present

Stage grading

Stage	TNM	% surviving 5 years		Surgical candidate?*
		Clinical staging	Surgical staging	
IA	T1N0M0	61	67	
IB	T2N0M0	38	57	
IIA	T1N1M0	34	55	
IIB	T2N1M0	24	39	Yes
	T3N0M0	22	38	
IIIA	T3N1M0	9	25	
	T1–3N2M0	13	23	
IIIB	T4N0–2M0	7	Not applicable	
	T1–4N3M0	3		No
IV	Any T, any NM1	1		

* One of the reasons why TNM stage grading is recommended is to accurately identify operable patients (identify anatomical extent of the disease) and avoid surgery in patients who have unresectable disease.

Diagnosis
• CXR ± CT scan to confirm suspicion
• Cytology: sputum, bronchoscopic brushing
• Biopsy: bronchoscopic for proximal lesions, percutaneous for peripheral lesions
• Pleural aspiration and biopsy for effusions
• Lymph node biopsy (needle aspiration or mediastinoscopy)
• Staging for metastasis: CT of the head and abdomen, skeletal-scintigraphy

Treatment

NSCLC:

- For stage I, II and IIIa, attempt curative surgery (± adjuvant chemotherapy or radiotherapy or neoadjuvant chemotherapy)
- For stage IIIb or IV: only palliative surgery

SCLC:

Treatment of extensive disease:

Majority of patients are diagnosed with incurable, extensive stage disease. Only ~ 5% of all patients with SCLC survive 5 years. Surgical resection is rarely considered. For most patients, the goal is symptom relief

- **Chemotherapy** is the standard treatment. ~ 80% of patients will respond to the treatment and ~ 20% respond completely. Median survival is ~ 9 months
- Since there is no benefit from maintenance chemotherapy, usually 4 - 6 cycles of **etoposide/cisplatin** are followed by observation
- Other chemotherapeutic drugs include: taxanes (paclitaxel [Taxol] and docetaxel), camptothecins (topotecan and irinotecan), gemcitabine, vinorelbine, cyclophosphamide

Treatment of limited disease:

- Combined chemotherapy and radiotherapy for the medically fit
- **Chemotherapy** is always included in the initial management (except in rare cases, when surgical resection is possible). **Cisplatin + etoposide** or **carboplatin + etoposide** (4 - 6 cycles) is a widely used regimen
- **Prophylactic cranial irradiation (PCI)** if complete response to induction therapy

BIBLIOGRAPHY

Sachs S, Fiore JJ: An overview of Lung Cancer, Respir Care Clin N Am 2003; 9: 1-25.

Yung RCW: Tissue diagnosis of Suspected Lung Cancer, Respir Care Clin N Am 2003; 9: 51-76.

Mountain CF: Revision in the International System for Staging Lung Cancer, Chest 1997; 111: 1710-1717.

17. Miscellaneous

17.1 Atelectasis

Definition
Collapsed alveoli or incomplete expansion of the lungs. Collapse may be local or diffuse. Atelectasis is one of the most common pulmonary complications after surgery and is also one of the most commonly seen abnormalities on CXR.

Etiology
Decreased lung expansion and risk factors:
- **Abdominal/thoracic surgery** often results in patient's ability to generate good lung expansion. Therefore, these patients are at high risk for developing postoperative atelectasis
- **Other precipitating conditions** that interfere with patient's ability to generate negative intrapleural pressure include: anesthesia, obesity, advanced age, chest wall deformities and pain
- Atelectasis may also be caused by: prolonged rest, persistent low V_T breathing, phrenic nerve damage, ↓ surfactant production (IRDS), airway obstruction with gas absorption, compression of parenchyma by PTX, tumor or pleural effusion and retained secretions

Clinical manifestations
- Breath sounds: ↓ or absent, ± crackles
- Percussion: dullness over affected area
- Rapid shallow breathing (tachypnea with hypopnea), dyspnea and use of accessory muscles with significant parenchymal involvement
- CXR = ↑ whiteout, elevated diaphragm and volume loss ipsilaterally and tracheal shift to affected side
- ↓ PaO_2 due to increased V/Q mismatch
- PFT = restrictive pattern with decreased FRC, V_C and lung compliance

Differential diagnosis
Bronchogenic carcinoma, spontaneous PTX, massive pleural effusion, lung abscess, pneumonia, diaphragmatic paralysis, pulmonary fibrosis, ascites and PE

Treatment
- With minimal postoperative atelectasis, walking, deep breathing and coughing should usually be sufficient to reverse the impairment

- In moderate atelectasis, lung expansion techniques such as incentive spirometry (IS) or positive expiratory pressure (PEP) therapy can help reverse or prevent atelectasis
- Bronchial hygiene therapy (i.e. chest physiotherapy) should be used when atelectasis is caused by excessive mucus or mucus plugs
- Oxygen for hypoxemia
- Mechanical ventilation with PEEP and high FIO_2 for severe cases to reinflate collapsed areas and support oxygenation until the patient gets better
- Fiberoptic bronchoscopy may be needed to treat obstructive atelectasis, i.e. to remove mucus plugs that obstruct large airways, resulting in airway obstruction and atelectasis distal to plugs

17.2 Hemoptysis

Definition

Hemoptysis is coughing up of blood from tracheobronchial tree or pulmonary parenchyma. Hematemesis is blood that originates from the stomach. Massive hemoptysis is defined as anywhere from 150 ml to 600 ml/24 hours. Massive hemoptysis is not common (< 5% of cases) but is potentially life-threatening and requires rapid evaluation and therapy. Common causes of massive hemoptysis include: TB, lung abscess, bronchiectasis, necrotizing pneumonia, mycetoma and trauma.

Hemoptysis	vs	Hematemesis
Bright red blood		Dark blood; food particles
Coughed up		Vomited
Alkaline pH		Acidic pH
Alveolar macrophages present		Alveolar macrophages not present
Sputum present		Sputum not present

Etiology

Common causes	Rare causes
Bronchogenic carcinoma	Trauma or iatrogenic (bronchoscopy, lung biopsy, PA
Chronic bronchitis	catheter, chest tube insertion)
(most common)	Mitral stenosis
Bronchiectasis	Foreign body aspiration
TB	Coagulopathy
Lung abscess	Goodpasture's syndrome
Bacterial pneumoni	Pulmonary AV fistula Wegener's granulomatosis
Cryptogenic fungal	PA aneurysm
infection (mycetoma)	Bronchiolithiasis
Pulmonary infarction	Sarcoidosis
	Bronchiolitis obliterans with organizing pneumonia
	Drug-induced: cocaine, thrombolytic agents, amiodarone

Diagnosis

- **History and physical examination:** confirm source; breath sounds and percussion may help localize site of pulmonary bleeding; examination of oro/nasopharynx (rhinoscopy and laryngoscopy) to rule out supraglottic bleeding; any history of epistaxis?
- **CXR:** patchy alveolar filling that becomes reticular over days; cavity; atelectasis or other abnormality likely to be related to the cause of hemoptysis
- **Bronchoscopy:** essential tool for visualizing and locating the source of bleeding. Fiberoptic bronchoscopy is used for small volumes of blood, while rigid bronchoscope is used with large volume hemoptysis. With massive hemoptysis, bronchoscopic evaluation is urgent; smaller hemoptysis should be investigated within 24 hours
- **CT:** allows detection of bronchiectasis, parenchymal nodules, cavities, infiltrates, endobronchial masses, vascular abnormalities, etc.

Treatment

Usually, hemoptysis requires no specific therapy. Treatment is directed at its underlying identified cause.

Treatment of massive hemoptysis

- **Endotracheal intubation** for airway control and to facilitate suctioning, ventilation/oxygenation and bronchoscopy

- **Rigid bronchoscopy:**
- Volume resuscitation (have IV in place), blood transfusion (get type and cross blood), coagulopathy correction
- If unilateral lung hemorrhage, protect good lung by:
  - Positioning 'presumed' bleeding side down (lateral decubitus position) so gravity will decrease the risk of blood entering the non-hemorrhagic lung
  - Use double-lumen ETT to allow unilateral ventilation and protection of good lung through cuffed bronchial lumen
- **Endobronchial tamponade** with balloon-tipped Fogarty catheter
- **Laser photocoagulation** is effective in controlling persistent hemoptysis due to airway carcinomas
- **Bronchial artery embolization** (guided by radiographic arteriography) may be used to occlude bronchial artery with embolizing material (e.g. polyvinyl alcohol) or **selective surgical resection** may be needed

17.3   Inhaled Poisons

17.3.1 Carbon monoxide (CO) poisoning

Definition
- Inspiring byproduct of fire (smoke, noxious gases, CO). Inhalation of CO leads to displacement of O_2 from binding sites on Hb
- CO combines with Hb ~ 210 x more strongly than
  O_2 = anemic hypoxia = tissue hypoxia

Incidence
~ 3500 - 4000 deaths/year in the USA

Clinical manifestations
Depend on the % of CO combined with Hb

COHb %	Signs/Symptoms
0 - 5%	None (normal value)
5 - 10%	Few minor complaints (e.g. visual impairment)
10 - 20%	Mild headache, tinnitus
20 - 30%	Severe headache, drowsiness, weakness
30 - 40%	Visual impairment, throbbing headache, nausea, vomiting

40 - 50%	Syncope, ↑ respiratory rate, ↑ heart rate, seizures, Cheyne - Stokes respirations
> 50 - 60%	Convulsions, shock, coma, death (COHb > 60 - 70%)

- Cherry red or pink skin is due to COHb formation, but is not reliable
- Pulse oximetry is of no value because it reads COHb as O_2; need to measure O_2 sat by direct co-oximetry
- ABG: ↑ COHb, metabolic acidosis; PaO_2 may be normal

Treatment
- High FIO_2: 100% O_2 until COHb deacreases to < 10%
- Hyperbaric chamber for severe CO poisoning (> 30 - 40%)
- Mechanical ventilation with COHb > 40 - 60%?

> **NOTE:** Half-life of COHb ~ 5 hours on room air, 90 min on 100% O_2, 23 min in hyperbaric chamber at 3 atm.

17.3.2 Cyanide poisoning

Severe cyanide poisoning has a very rapid onset and occurs in some cases of smoke inhalation. Increased risk in individuals exposed to smoke generated from combustion of plastics and polyurethanes. Cyanide blocks oxidative phosphorylation and mitochondrial O_2 utilization, which ⇒ lactic acidosis. Survival may be associated with anoxic brain damage.

Clinical features
- Anxiety, headache, nausea, dizziness, tachycardia, tachypnea, dyspnea
- Pink skin and mucous membranes
- Unexplained metabolic acidosis
- Convulsions, apnea, seizures
- Smell of bitter almonds (not reliable)
- Venous blood hyperoxygenation

Treatment
- Administer high O_2%; if necessary, intubate and ventilate with 100% O_2
- Start IV line and cardiac monitoring

- Cyanide antidotes:
  - **Amyl nitrate** is recommended as an initial temporary measure for non-medical person to administer in the form of inhalation. The ampule is broken and contents are emptied onto a cloth; this is held to mouth/nose of the patient to be inhaled until IV access is obtained for administration of sodium nitrate
  - **Sodium nitrate** 0.33 ml/kg of 3% solution IV (not > 10 ml); induces HbMet formation and vasodilation
  - **Sodium thiosulfate (Tinver)** 12.5 g (50 ml) IV at 3 - 5 ml/min as a 2nd line therapy
  - **Dicobalt (Kelocyanor)** 300 mg IV over 1 min followed by 50 ml of 50% glucose (dextrose); may repeat after 5 min if no response; caution: dicobalt is severely toxic in the absence of cyanide (avoid if possible)

17.4   The Lung in Adverse Environments

17.4.1   Altitude sickness

Introduction to high altitude

- Normal sea level Pb of 760 mmHg is **halved** at 5500 m (18,000 ft):
  recall alveolar air equation: $PaO_2 = (Pb - PH_2O) \times FIO_2 - (PaCO_2 - R)$.
  Therefore, $\uparrow$ **altitude** $\Rightarrow \downarrow$ Pb $\Rightarrow \downarrow PaO_2$. Basically, PaO_2 will $\downarrow$ by ~ ½ its value at sea level every 5500 m in altitude. At 8850 m (29,028 ft) (Mt. Everest), the atmospheric pressure is about 250 mmHg, which $\Rightarrow PaO_2$ of ~ 40 - 45 mmHg
- Respiratory system compensates for hypoxemia secondary to high altitude ($\downarrow$ Pb) by:
  - $\uparrow$ **ventilation:** $PaO_2 < 60$ mmHg stimulates peripheral chemoreceptors to send signals to medulla to $\uparrow$ ventilation
  - **Polycythemia:** hormone erythropoietin from kidney stimulates RBC production by bone marrow ($\uparrow$ Hb = $\uparrow O_2$ carrying capacity); also seen in patients with chronic hypoxemia (COPD, heart failure)

(1) Acute Mountain Sickness (AMS)

Most common altitude-related illness. It is unusual at altitudes < 2500 meters

Symptoms:

Occur when ascent to altitude is too rapid; most people experience symptoms when ascend to > 3000 m (10,000 ft). Symptoms may appear immediately or 2 - 3 days after arrival at high altitude:

- Headache, dyspnea, irritation
- Anorexia, nausea or vomiting
- Fatigue or weakness, ± peripheral edema
- Dizziness or lightheadedness
- Difficulty sleeping

Management:
- Usually self-limiting. Prevention: slow, gradual ascent or descend 300 - 900 m (1000 - 3000 ft) when experience symptoms
- **Acetazolamide (Diamox)** 250 mg q6 h or for prevention: 125 - 250 mg bid starting 1 day before ascent and continuing for ≥ 2 days at altitude
- **Dexamethasone** 2 - 4 mg PO q6 h for prevention and treatment (usually not needed)
- Portable hyperbaric bag to simulate descent to lower altitude is usually needed only if AMS is complicated by high altitude pulmonary edema or high altitude cerebral edema

(2) High Altitude Pulmonary Edema (HAPE)

Description:
- HAPE is less common than AMS but is the most common cause of death related to high altitude. It is a noncardiogenic pulmonary edema of unknown etiology; possibly due to hypoxia-induced pulmonary vasoconstriction ⇒ ↑ capillary permeability ⇒ ↑ ↑ pulmonary artery pressure and leakage into alveoli
- May be fatal within a few hours if not treated by descent and/or oxygen

Clinical features:
- Initial symptoms: dry cough, dyspnea at rest or exertion, chest tightness, fatigue and weakness, followed by productive cough, tachycardia, tachypnea, crackles, cyanosis, ± pink and frothy sputum
- CXR: of use for high-altitude clinic or hospital. Patchy, fluffy infiltrates are seen

Management:
- **Descent/evacuation** to lower altitude and **oxygen** 4 - 6 L/min if available. Often, a descent of ~ 300 - 900 m ⇒ significant improvement
- **Nifedipine (Procardia, Adalat)** 10 mg PO q6 h; then 20 - 30 mg slow-release PO bid
- **Portable hyperbaric bag** (e.g. Gamow bag), if available, for temporary treatment before descent is achieved

(3) High Altitude Cerebral Edema (HACE)

Description:

Lower incidence than HAPE. Occurs occasionally in conjunction with HAPE. It is rapidly fatal if untreated and the management and prevention are similar to that of HAPE

Signs and symptoms:

- Headache, nausea, vomiting, disorientation
- Seizures, severe lassitude, changes in level of consciousness
- Cyanosis, retinal hemorrhage, hallucinations
- If untreated, patient may become unconscious and die

Management:

- **Prompt descent** to lower altitude and **oxygen** if available
- **Dexamethasone** 4 mg IM, IV or PO, followed by 4 mg q6 h thereafter; helps ↓ cerebral edema and should be used while waiting for evacuation
- **Portable hyperbaric bag** if available

BIBLIOGRAPHY

Barry PW, Pollard AJ: Altitude Illness, BMJ 2003; 326: 915-920.

Harris MD et al: High-altitude Medicine, Am Fam Physician 1998; 57: 1907 - 1914.

Hackett PH, Roach RC: High-altitude Illness, N Engl J Med 2001; 345: 107-114.

17.4.2 Diving injuries

(1) Barotrauma/Air Gas Embolism
- For every 10 m (33 ft) descent below sea level, pressure increases to 1 atm (760 mmHg). Pressure at 20 m (66 ft) = 3 atm (2280 mmHg). Example: inhaling to TLC of 6 L and diving to 10 m = lungs compress to ~ 3 L; 20 m to ~ 2 L; and 30 m ~ 1.5 L
- During ascent, the diver must continually exhale in order to allow expanding compressed air in the lungs to escape. If the intrathoracic gas volume overexpands (e.g. rapid ascent), alveolar septae will rupture and expanding gas may enter mediastinum (**mediastinal emphysema**) and pleural space (**PTX**). Mediastinal gas may further expand into pericardial sac or subcutaneous tissues of the neck (**subcutaneous emphysema**). If expanding alveolar gas enters pulmonary veins, it will form a potentially life-threatening **air gas embolism**

(2) Decompression Sickness
If ascent is too rapid, gases are released from tissues as bubbles which can cause joint pains, chest pain, paresthesia and paralysis and death if severe
↑ Risk: old age, obesity, dehydration, alcohol use, exercise, unpressurized flight after dive, caisson workers

Signs and symptoms:
- **Bends:** occur within minutes to within a few hours after ascent and are due to bubbles causing vascular occlusion. Characterized by deep pain in large joints, most commonly hips, elbows and knees
- **Chokes:** cough, substernal burning chest pain and breathlessness without hemodynamic collapse. It is thought that ↑ pulmonary artery and RV pressures ± ↑ interstitial fluid play a major role. Most commonly seen immediately after decompression
- **Skin mottling, rash (pruritus):** 'skin bends' cause itching of the skin; often disappear within a few hours
- **Spinal cord decompression sickness:** probably most dangerous symptom, which is characterized by ascending parasthesias and paralysis and is often associated with bowel and bladder dysfunction. Most cases occur within 1 - 2 hours after an exposure

Management:

Treatment of air gas embolism and decompression sickness is similar. The mainstay of therapy is decompression to shrink bubbles and increase the pressure gradient to drive gas back into solution. Prevention: slow ascent and staged 'decompression' periods with deep dives.

- 100% oxygen, intubate and perform cardiopulmonary resuscitation (CPR) if needed
- Do not place in Trendelenburg position
- Contact closest hyperbaric facility and transport the patient; helicopter must fly at < 300 m (~ 1000 ft) or, if using airplane, cabin must be pressurized to 1 atm
- The following may be of benefit: corticosteroids, lidocaine, aspirin?
  (if no active bleeding)

BIBLIOGRAPHY

Neuman TS: Arterial Gas Embolism and Decompression Sickness, News Physiol Sci 2002; 17: 77-81.

Bellini LS, Grippi MA: Diving Injuries and Air Embolism. In, Fishman AP et al: Fishman's Manual of Pulmonary Diseases and Disorders, 3rd ed. McGraw-Hill, 2002.

18. Neonatal and Pediatric Disorders

18.1 Bronchiolitis

Definition
- Inflammation, swelling and constriction of bronchioles secondary to viral infection
- Usually affects children < 2 years of age

Etiology
- RSV causes ~ 75% of all cases
- Also: parainfluenza and other viruses

Clinical manifestations
- **Signs and symptoms:** cough, nasal discharge, dyspnea, retractions, wheezing, rhonchi or crackles, hypoxemia
- CXR: hyperinflation $\pm$ infiltrates

Treatment
- Many cases are self-limiting, with need only of supportive care
- If without respiratory distress, treat at home: nasal saline drops, humidity, suction with bulb
- If hospitalized:
  - Humidified O_2 30 - 40% via hood in most cases
  - Suction
  - Isolation
  - Hydration
  - Bronchodilators
  - Steroids?
  - **RSV-immune globulin intravenously (RespiGam)** to $\downarrow$ incidence of RSV in high-risk patients (BPD or premature birth)
  - **Ribavirin?** (if severe, via small particle aerosol generator (SPAG) nebulizer for 12 - 18 hours/day for 3 - 7 days; NOT as effective as previously thought; MV for RF)

18.2 Bronchopulmonary Dysplasia (BPD)

Definition/Etiology
Lung injury secondary to prolonged use of: mechanical ventilation, high FIO_2, high PIP; most common in low birthweight (LBW) and RDS infants (premature lungs); leads to mucosal hyperplasia, thick secretions and fibrosis = $\downarrow$ diffusion across

A-C membrane; ↑ risk: immaturity with LBW (< 1.5 kg), gestational age < 34 weeks, ↑ duration of O_2 and PPV, infection

Clinical manifestations

↑ RR and HR; retractions; persistent cyanosis; grunting; crackles/wheeze; PH.
CXR: overinflation (hyperlucency), 'ground-glass' appearance; hypoxemia/hypercapnia; failure to thrive; PTX, PIE may complicate BPD resulting from high P_{peak} and ↓ CL

Treatment

Supportive; O_2; MV with low PIP, mean airway pressure, (PEEP to ↓ FIO_2 levels); diuretics and digitalis for RHF; bronchodilators: β_2-agonist, theophylline (to ↑ diaphragm contractility); steroids? to control inflammation

18.3   Croup and Epiglottitis

	Croup (laryngotracheobronchitis)	Epiglottitis
Definition	Inflammation of subglottic area (vocal cord involvement)	Inflammation of epiglottis ⇒ edema and possibly life-threatening complete airway obstruction!
Etiology	**Parainfluenza virus** is No.1 cause (≥ 75%); also, RSV, influenza virus	No.1 cause: *H. influenza* type B bacteria (↓ incidence since invention of Hib vaccine in 1980s)
Clinical features		
Age	3 months - 5 years	3 - 7 years
Onset	Gradual: 2 - 3 days	Acute: within hours
Cough	Barking (seal-like)	Minimal
Voice	Hoarseness	Muffled
Stridor	Yes	Yes
Fever	Low-grade	High (≥ 39°C)
Drooling	No	Yes (secondary to dysphagia)
WBC	Normal (viral infection)	↑ (bacterial infect)
Retractions	+/-	Yes

↑ HR, RR	Yes	Yes
Diagnosis	'steeple sign' on lateral neck X-ray confirms diagnosis; (subglottic narrowing = haziness) Confirmed by lateral neck X-ray (supraglottic haziness)	Performed only after intubation. Visualized by depressing the tongue with a tongue blade or direct laryngoscopy: shows cherry-red swollen epiglottis; should only be performed in the operating room by experienced intubator (touching epiglottis may ⇒ spasm ⇒ complete obstruction!)
Treatment	• No stridor at rest (only on exertion): = mild obstruction; patient can be treated at home with cool mist	• **Establish airway** (intubation or tracheotomy) until inflammation resolves; usually can extubate in ≤ 3 days, when air leak can be heard around ETT when bagging
Treatment	• Stridor at rest: hospitalize and give: ○ Humidified O_2 (30 - 40%) via mist tent ○ **Racemic epinephrine** nebulized (0.25 - 0.5 ml of 2.25% solution) diluted in 3 ml NS qid or 0.05 ml/kg/ dose diluted in 3 ml NS (max 0.5 ml) ○ **Dexamethasone** IM or PO ○ Budesonide (respules) nebulized	**Antibiotics**, hydration, humidified O_2 by blow-by • MV if paralyzation is required: low PIP, RR and FIO_2 usually, as lung is healthy • Steroids and racemic epinephrine are ineffective

Epiglottitis patient will usually be in more distress ('toxic appearance') compared with croup patient and will be irritable, complain of sore throat (if able) and adopt 'tripod-position', with head/neck extended forward in an attempt to get more air in.

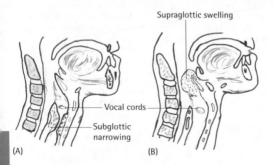

Fig. 31　Figure A: Croup (swollen tracheal tissue). Figure B: Epiglottitis (swollen epiglottis)

18.4　Cystic Fibrosis (CF)

Definition

Inherited autosomal recessive disease. It is the most common lethal genetic disease in white people. Autosomal recessive mutation occurs on chromosome 7, to the gene coding for the CF transmembrane conductance regulator (CFTR), which acts as a chloride channel. This leads to altered chloride and water transport in cells, high Na^+ and Cl^- concentrations in sweat test and exocrine gland malfunction, which increases mucus viscosity. 1:25 white people are carriers, which means that there is a 25% chance that a child will have CF if both parents carry the CF gene.

Clinical features

- Meconium ileus (distal intestinal obstruction): failure to pass meconium in the 1st 12 - 24 hours of life. This occurs in ~ 5 - 10% of CF patients
- Pancreatic insufficiency: steatorrhea, failure to thrive, malnutrition
- Recurrent pneumonia, upper respiratory tract infections and bronchiectasis
- Dyspnea, decreased exercise tolerance, clubbing
- Cough with large amounts of thick sputum, ± hemoptysis
- Hypoxemia and hypercarbia
- CXR: hyperinflation; ↑ A-P diameter; ↓ volume

Diagnosis
- In > 90% of prenatal screening, diagnosis is possible
- Sweat Cl⁻ test > 60 mEq/l in children

Treatment
- Antibiotics for infections: most common childhood pathogen is *Staphylococcus*, then *Pseudomonas*
- Inhaled antibiotics for *Pseudomonas aeruginosa*:
  - **Tobramycin** (TOBI; 300 mg twice/day)
  - **Colistin** (Coly-Mycin): 150 mg twice/day as alternative to TOBI
- **Pulmozyme** (rhDNase) nebulized to decrease mucus thickness
- Oxygen, bronchodilators
- Airway clearance techniques:
  - Chest physiotherapy: postural drainage (PD), percussion, vibration
  - PEP: patient exhales against resistance of ~ 10 - 20 cmH$_2$O to keep airway open and mobilize secretions. MDI or nebulizer can be used together with PEP device to administer aerosolized treatments
  - Flutter device (vibrating PEP): to loosen up secretions for easier coughing up; patient takes a deep breath, holds it for ~ 3 seconds and, with flutter device in mouth, exhales fully. During exhalation, the ball in the device bounces, which causes vibrations of secretions in the airways, making it easier for the patient to cough them up
- Nutrition: increase calories, water, carbohydrates and protein. Pancreatic enzymes, vitamin supplementation (A, D, E, K) ± feeding via NG or gastrostomy tube

Prognosis
Median survival age ~ 30 years

18.5   Infant Respiratory Distress Syndrome (IRDS)

Definition/Etiology: (aka hyaline membrane disease–HMD)
- Secondary to surfactant deficiency and immature lungs which ⇒ alveolar collapse at end-expiration and ↓ lung volumes
- ↑ Risk: maternal diabetes mellitus (DM), Cesarean-section, fetal asphyxia, 2nd twin, 3rd trimester bleed. IRDS usually occurs in infants < 35 weeks' gestation and LBW

Clinical manifestations
- Low Apgar score
- Nasal flaring
- Grunting with or without stethoscope

- Marked retractions
- Cyanosis
- Refractory hypoxemia
- ↓ BS with crackles
- CXR: ↓ volume with 'ground glass' - reticulogranular or honeycomb appearance
- Lecithin/sphyngomyelin (L/S) ratio < 2 = ↑ risk for IRDS

Treatment

- PaO_2 should be > 50 - 70 mmHg (use oxyhood initially?)
- CPAP at 3 - 5 cmH$_2$O for moderate hypoxemia and vigorous infant
- Intubate/ventilator for RF:
  - $PaCO_2$ > 55 mmHg, PaO_2 < 50 mmHg on FIO_2 > 0.6
  - Initial settings: PIP 20 - 25 cmH$_2$O; PEEP 5 cmH$_2$O; RR 40 - 60/min; FIO_2 0.40 - 1.0; inspiratory time (Ti) ≤ 0.4 sec
- **Prevention: Steroids** (betamethasone or dexamethasone) to mother ~ 48 hours prior to premature delivery to stimulate neonatal surfactant production and thus ↓ risk of IRDS or its severity
- **Surfactant administration:** (i.e. Survanta, Exosurf) immediately after birth for prevention or ~ 6 - 8 hours after birth for rescue treatment (see chapter on Respiratory Drugs for more information on surfactants). For all infants < 1.3 kg or < 32-week gestation age

18.6 Meconium Aspiration Syndrome (MAS)

Definition

- Aspiration of meconium (green material = 1st newborn stool) in utero or during initial breaths secondary to asphyxia
- Often seen in full-term and post-term (> 43 weeks) newborns
- May lead to:
  - Obstructed airways ⇒ air trapping secondary to 'ball-valve' obstruction; patient is able to inspire but on expiration, airways close
  - PPHN
  - Chemical pneumonitis
  - Hypoxemia

Etiology

- ↑ Risk: maternal DM, smoking, oligohydramnios

NOTE: *Newborns with thin watery meconium are less likely to have severe respiratory problems compared with those with thick 'green pea soup' meconium.*

Clinical manifestations
- Signs and symptoms: low Apgar score, gasping respirations, grunting, retractions, tachypnea, cyanosis, nasal flaring, crackles with decreased air entry
- CXR: hyperinflation, diffuse patchy infiltrate and ↓ aeration (atelectasis)
- ABG: hypoxemia, hypercarbia, mixed acidosis

Treatment
- **At head delivery**, suction oropharynx with bulb before infant initiates 1st breath. Place newborn on preheated radiant warmer. If meconium is thin, respiratory problems are usually not severe. **If meconium is thick**, intubate and apply direct suction to ETT, extubate, reintubate and repeat suction until no meconium (use 100% O_2 blow-by throughout procedure) is left
- **NB:** DO NOT BMV until all meconium is suctioned, if possible, as it may be forced into lower airways
- O_2 via hood
- CPAP
- Mechanical ventilation when: pH < 7.20, $PaCO_2$ > 70 mmHg, PaO_2 < 50 mmHg, SpO_2 < 90%
  Settings: short Ti and long Te to ↓ air trapping; lowest P_{peak} to achieve good chest excursion and adequate V_T

18.7 Persistent Pulmonary Hypertension of the Newborn (PPHN)

Definition
- Pulmonary HTN (↑ PVR) secondary to heart or lung disease
- aka persistent fetal circulation (PFC)

Etiology
- ↓ PaO_2 ⇒ vasoconstriction of pulmonary vessels ⇒ PH
- High risk with: MAS, IRDS, CDH, sepsis, pneumonia, CHF

Clinical manifestations
- Refractory hypoxemia
- Possibly no distress at birth
- Tachypnea with periods of apnea
- Cyanosis

Diagnosis

- Preductal (right radial) $PaO_2 \sim$ 15 - 20 mmHg > postductal
  (left radial or umbilical artery)
- Preductal and postductal SpO_2 can help in identifying R - L shunt across ductus arteriosus (DA):
  - Example: preductal SpO_2 = 95% and postductal (left lower leg)
    SpO_2 = 79%
- Pulmonary hypertension

Treatment

- Hyperventilation to achieve: $PaCO_2$ 25 - 30 mmHg, pH $\geq$ 7.50, alkalosis
  = ↓ pulmonary vasoconstriction
- **Nitric oxide** (pulmonary vasodilator)
  - ↓ PVR, PAP and R - L shunt = ↑ PaO_2
  - Delivered through inspiratory side of ventilator circuit at ~ 20 ppm (parts per million)
- **Tolazoline:** vasodilates pulmonary vascular bed to ↓ PVR and PAP;
  Caution: side effects of systemic hypotension
- Oxygen
- Volume expanders, dobutamine and dopamine, may be used to offset hypotension and R - L shunt

18.8 Congenital Diaphragmatic Hernia (CDH)

Definition/Etiology

- Abdominal contents enter thorax as a result of undeveloped diaphragm (85% occur on left side, through foramen of Bochdalek)
- Abdominal contents compress lungs; this may lead to atelectasis, hypoxemia and hypoplasia of ipsilateral lung

Signs and symptoms

- Respiratory distress unresponsive to O_2 or BMV with PPV
- ↓/absent BS or bowel sounds heard on affected side
- Scaphoid (sunken) abdomen
- CXR confirms diagnosis: abdominal organs in thorax, mediastinal shift away from affected side (can be detected prenatally by ultrasound)

Treatment
- NG tube to ↓ gastric distention
- **NB:** DO NOT BMV: intubate and MV if necessary to ventilate; if suspect CDH at birth, intubate to prevent air from entering stomach and compressing lungs
- O_2
- Prompt surgery
- HFV? ECMO?

18.9   Other Disorders

18.9.1   Apnea of prematurity (AOP)

No breathing for > 20 s + cyanosis, ↓ HR, ↓ muscle tone. Apneic spells are usually related to gestational age

Etiology

Multifactorial causes: brainstem immaturity, various cardiopulmonary diseases/anomalies, CNS dysfunction

Treatment

Treat the cause; monitor for apnea in < 35 week gestational age (monitor at home with impedance pneumogram); tactile stimulation; theophylline for frequent spells; nasal CPAP at 3 - 5 cmH_2O if theophylline ineffective; ventilatory support if severe

18.9.2   Choanal atresia

Partial or complete blockage of nasopharynx secondary to membrane tissue. If unilateral, may be asymptomatic or mild respiratory distress. If bilateral ⇒ asphyxia; respiratory emergency because neonates are obligate nose breathers

Clinical manifestations

Gasping, retractions, cyanosis with initial breaths, apnea

Diagnosis

Failure to pass catheter (e.g. 6 Fr catheter) through infant's nose

Treatment

Insert oral airway if bilateral to establish mouth breathing ± intubate; if no response to oral airway, surgical correction (puncture membrane) is the ultimate management

18.9.3   Foreign body aspiration

Most aspirated objects lodge in right main stem bronchus

Etiology

Commonly aspirated objects: seed, peanut, grape, hot dog
(highest risk: 6 months - 4 years of age)

Clinical manifestations

Coughing; gagging; dyspnea; cyanosis; BS: ↓, absent or unilateral wheezing; many
aspirated objects are radiolucent and may not be seen on CXR: inspiratory and
expiratory films may help in locating area of air trapping

Treatment

Heimlich maneuver, rigid bronchoscopy (or flexible), bronchodilators, CPT

18.9.4   Pierre - Robin syndrome (PRS)

Micrognathia (small jaw) ± glossoptosis (downward tongue) ⇒ ↑ risk of airway
obstruction as a result of the tongue being more posterior than normal

Clinical manifestations

Retractions if severe; choking with feeding (usually by age 6 months, feeding
problems decrease, as mandible grows to its appropriate size)

Treatment

Prone position while sleeping to ↓ risk of airway obstruction; feed by NG tube;
tongue surgery (to hold in place); tracheostomy if life-threatening airway
obstruction

18.9.5   Retinopathy of prematurity (ROP)

Formation of scar tissue behind lens, causing partial or full blindness

Etiology

High PO_2, rather than FIO_2: retinal vessels constrict as a result of hyperoxia ⇒ vessel
necrosis; vessels proliferate in order to reestablish blood supply to retina; vessels may
hemorrhage, resulting in scar tissue behind retina, which may detach; ↑ risk with:
prematurity, high PO_2, ↓ birth weight, ↓ gestational age

Treatment

Maintain PO_2 50 - 80 mmHg and SaO_2 < 97%; cryosurgery: probe cooled with nitrous
oxide to - 20°C is introduced behind the eye, avascular part of retina is frozen,

preventing further vessel proliferation; laser surgery: laser photocoagulates avascular part of retina (less invasive and traumatic than cryosurgery)

18.9.6 Transient tachypnea of the newborn (TTNB)

Respiratory distress at birth as a result of delayed absorption of lung fluid at birth

Etiology
Predisposing factors: Cesarean section, epidural hypotension, asphyxia, maternal DM, prolapsed cord, excessive oxytocin in labor

Clinical manifestations
Tachypnea as high as 150/min, retractions, grunting, nasal flaring, cyanosis, good Apgar score at birth, but within hours respiratory distress develops (usually resolves in ≤ 3 days, while IRDS does not)

Treatment
Usually self-limiting within 3 days; O_2 hood 30 - 50% to maintain PO_2 50 - 70 mmHg, CPAP if no response to O_2 alone, ventilatory support is usually not needed

BIBLIOGRAPHY

American Thoracic Society: Guidelines for the Management of Adults with Community-acquired Pneumonia: Diagnosis, Assessment of Severity, Antimicrobial Therapy and Prevention, Am J Respir Crit Care Med 2001; 163: 1730-1754.

American Thoracic Society/Center for Disease Control and Prevention/ Infectious Society of America Official Joint Statement: Treatment of Tuberculosis, Am J Respir Crit Care Med 2003; 167: 603-662.

American Thoracic Society: Hospital-acquired Pneumonia in Adults: Diagnosis, Assessment of Severity, Initial Antimicrobial Therapy and Prevention Strategies: A Consensus Statement. Am J Respir Crit Care Med 1996; 153: 1711-1725.

American Thoracic Society: Idiopathic Pulmonary Fibrosis: Diagnosis and Treatment: International Consensus Statement, Am J Respir Crit Care Med 2000; 161: 646-664.

American Thoracic Society: Statement on Sarcoidosis, Am J Respir Crit Care Med 1999; 160: 736-755.

Albert RK, Spiro SG, Jett JR: Comprehensive Respiratory Medicine, Mosby, 1999.

Barnhart SL, Czervinske MP: Perinatal and Pediatric Respiratory Care, WB Saunders, 2003.

Chapman SW et al: Practice Guidelines for the Management of Patients with Blastomycosis. Infectious Disease Society of America. Clin Infect Dis 2000; 30: 679-683.

DesJardins T, Burton GG: Clinical Manifestations and Assessment of Respiratory Disease, 4th ed. Mosby, 2002.

Expert Panel Report 2: Guidelines for the Diagnosis and Management of Asthma. National Asthma Education and Prevention Program, National Heart, Lung and Blood Institute, National Institutes of Health. Bethesda, Maryland: Publication No. 97-4053, 1997 and Updates NAEPP Expert Panel Report 2 on selected topics, Publication No. 97-4051, 2002.

Fishman AP et al: Fishman's Manual of Pulmonary Diseases and Disorders, 3rd ed. McGraw Hill, 2002.

Galgiani JN et al: Practice Guidelines for the Treatment of Coccidoidomycosis. Infectious Disease Society of America. Clin Infect Dis 2000; 30: 658-661.

Ghofrani HA et al: Sildenafil for Treatment of Lung Fibrosis and Pulmonary Hypertension: A Randomized Controlled Trial. Lancet, 2002; 360: 895-900.

Global Initiative for Chronic Obstructive Lung Disease (GOLD), Executive Summary: Global strategy for the diagnosis, management and prevention of COPD, updated July 2003. (Based on April 1998 NHLBI/WHO Workshop) www.goldcopd.com

Grossman RF, Fein A: Evidence-based Assessment of Diagnostic Tests for Ventilator-associated Pneumonia: Executive Summary. Chest 2000; 117: 177-181.

Johns MW: A New Method for Measuring Daytime Sleepiness: The Epworth Sleepiness Scale. Sleep 1991; 14: 540-545.

Lynch JP III: Hospital-acquired Pneumonia: Risk Factors, Microbiology and Treatment. Chest 2001; 119: 373-384.

Saag MS et al: Practice Guidelines for the Management of Cryptococcal Disease. Infectious Disease Society of America. Clin Infect Dis 2000; 30: 710-718.

Singer M, Webb A: Oxford Handbook of Critical Care. Oxford University Press, 1997.

Stevens DA et al: Practice Guidelines for Diseases Caused by Aspergillus. Infectious Disease Society of America. Clin Infect Dis 2000; 30: 696-709.

Rubin LJ et al: Bosentan Therapy for Pulmonary Artery Hypertension, N Engl J Med 2002; 346: 896-903.

Wilkens H et al: Effect of Inhaled Iloprost Plus Oral Sildenafil in Patients with Primary Pulmonary Hypertension, Circulation 2001; 104: 1218.

Weinberger SE: Principles of Pulmonary Medicine, 4th ed. WB Saunders, 2004.

West JB: Pulmonary Physiology and Pathophysiology, LWW, 2001.

Wheat J et al: Practice Guidelines for the Management of Patients with Histoplasmosis. Infectious Disease Society of America. Clin Infect Dis 2000; 30: 688-695.

Whitaker K: Comprehensive Perinatal and Pediatric Respiratory Care, 3rd ed. Delmar Publishers, 2001.

THERAPEUTICS

19. Respiratory Drugs

19.1 Bronchodilators (BDs)

Agent	Dose	Action	Notes
Adrenergic agents (Sympathomimetics) **MA:** stimulate β_2- receptors $\Rightarrow$ activation of 3',5' cAMP $\Rightarrow$ relaxation of airway smooth muscle **AE:** tremors, palpitations, mild hypertension, tachycardia, tolerance if excessive, excessive use $\Rightarrow$ $\downarrow$ K^+ $\Rightarrow$ arrhythmias			
Albuterol [Proventil, Ventolin]	Neb: 2.5 mg in 3 ml NS tid, qid MDI: 90 µg/puff; 2 puffs q4 - 6 h DPI: 200 µg cap; q4 - 6 h Tab: 2 mg, 4 mg, tid, qid (extended release tab 4 mg, 8 mg, q12 h) Ped: 1.25 - 2.5 mg/dose via neb Infant: 0.1 mg/kg/dose NB: 0.1 - 0.5 mg/kg/dose q2 - 6 h	$\beta_2 > \beta 1$ onset: 15 min duration: 3 - 6 h	Currently most favored selective β_2 agonist. May mix with Atrovent or Cromolyn
Bitolterol [Tornalate]	Neb: 1.25 ml (0.2%) in 2.5 ml NS bid, tid, qid MDI: 2 puffs q8 h (0.37 mg/puff)	$\beta_2 > \beta 1$ onset: 3 min duration: 5 - 8 h	NOT used often. **Prodrug** hydrolyzed over time by esterases in lungs into **colterol**

Epinephrine [Adrenalin]	Neb: 0.25 - 0.50 ml in 2.5 ml NS MDI: 1 - 2 puffs (0.2 mg/puff) SC: 0.1 - 0.3 mg of 1:1,000 solution	α, β onset: 3 - 5 min duration: 1 - 3 h	NOT used often. High adverse effects due to strong β_1 effects. May be useful in acute asthma and hypersensitivity reactions
Formoterol [Foradil]	DPI: 1 puff bid (12 µg, 60/pack)	onset: < 3 min duration: 12 h	NOT for acute bronchospasm. Long-acting BD for maintenance therapy (similar to salmeterol but very quick onset)
Isoetharine [Bronkosol]	Neb: 0.25 - 0.50 ml in 3 ml NS q4 h	onset: < 5 min duration: 1 - 3 h	NOT used often. Inactivated by heat, light, air - turns **pink**: discard (sputum may tinge pink)
Isoproterenol [Isuprel]	Neb: 2.5 - 5 mg/dose in 2.5 ml NS	onset: < 5 min duration: 0.5 - 3 h	NOT used often due to its AE (strong β_1), short duration and availability of better BDs
Levalbuterol [Xopenex]	Neb: > 12 years: 0.63 or 1.25 mg in 3 ml q6 - 8 h	Strong β_2 onset: 15 min duration: 5 - 8 h	Racemic form of albuterol Less β_1 than albuterol = ↓ AE + ↑ duration
Metaproterenol [Alupent]	Neb: 0.2 - 0.3 ml in 2.5 ml NS q4 h MDI: 2 - 3 puffs q3 - 4 h	Weak β_1, mild β_2 onset: < 5 min duration: 2 - 4 h	
Pirbuterol [Maxair]	MDI: 2 puffs q4 - 6 h (0.2 mg/puff)	$\beta_2 > \beta_1$ onset: 5 min duration: 3 - 5 h	

Racemic epinephrine [Vapo-, Micro-, or Asthmanefrin]	Neb: 0.25 - 0.50 ml of 2.25% sol in 3 ml NS	α and β onset: 5 min duration: 0.5 - 2 h	Mainly used as topical **vasoconstrictor** for stridor resulting from croup and laryngeal edema
Salmeterol [Serevent]	MDI: 2 puffs bid (21 μg/puff)	β_2 onset: 20 min duration: 12 h	NOT for acute bronchospasm. Long-acting BD for maintenance therapy of asthma
Terbutaline [Brethine, Bricanyl]	Neb: 0.25 mg in 2.5 ml NS q4 - 6 h MDI: 2 puffs q4 - 6 h Tab: 2.5, 5 mg tid	$\beta_2 > \beta1$ onset: 5 - 15 min duration: 3 - 6 h	Used also for **tocolysis** - inhibition of premature labor (relaxes uterine smooth muscle)

Anticholinergic agents (Parasympatholytics):
MA: inhibit smooth muscle contraction by blocking muscarinic receptors to ↓ cGMP and Ach release. Also, ↓ mucus secretion.
AE: dry mouth, blurred vision, cough
Caution: in patients with glaucoma, prostatic hypertrophy or bladder obstruction

Ipratropium [Atrovent]	Neb: 1 unit dose vial (0.5 mg in 2.5 ml) usually mixed with albuterol. MDI: 2 puffs qid	onset: 5 - 15 min duration: 4 - 6 h	Used for maintenance therapy for bronchospasm in COPD patients ± asthma. Also comes premixed with albuterol for neb **(DuoNeb)** and MDI **(Combivent)**

Atropine		onset: 15 min duration: 3 - 4 h	**NOT** used any more as BD due to its AE such as: ↑ mucus thickness, blurred vision, ↑ HR, hallucinations, etc.
Tiotropium [Spiriva]	DPI: 1 inh/d (18 µg/inh)	onset: 30 min duration: 24 h	**NOT** approved yet in USA (8/2003)

Methylxanthines:

MA: not clear; inhibit phosphodiesterase ⇒ ↑ cAMP ⇒ bronchial smooth muscle relaxation. There are other theories

EF: ↑ diaphragm contraction, ↑ mucociliary action, ↑ resp center drive, ↑ CO, +ve inotropic and chronotropic effect, ↑ myocardial muscle perfusion, ↓ PVR, ↑ diuresis

AE: has narrow therapeutic dose (5 - 15 µg/ml); toxicity with > 20 µg/ml: seizure, nausea, arrhythmia, diarrhea, convulsions, irritability, hyperglycemia

| Aminophylline [Theophylline] | <u>Adults:</u> Load: 6 mg/kg IVMaintenance: 0.5 - 0.7 mg/kg/h IV inf <u>Neonate:</u> 0.2 mg/kg/h | Weak BD at therapeutic levels. May be of use for COPD ± asthma patients due to its other effects | Used as maintenance drug in COPD due to its bronchodilating and nonbroncho-dilating effects (see EF above); Adjunct to mod-severe asthma; infant apnea (also caffeine) |

19.2 Corticosteroids (CS)

Corticosteroids are potent anti-inflammatory drugs. They are mainly used for asthma and acute exacerbation of COPD. Other uses include: sarcoidosis and other ILDs, chemical pneumonitis, cancer (CA), rheumatoid arthritis and for mothers delivering premature infants, in order to stimulate the baby's surfactant production and ↓ IRDS risk.

Inhaled corticosteroids:

MA: help alleviate airway obstruction by: ↓ inflammation, ↑ β_2 agonist responsiveness and ↓/prevent hypersensitivity reactions

EF: 6 - 12 h into therapy (NOT for acute asthma attack)

AE: using inhaled steroids ⇒ ↓ AE of systemic steroids (see systemic corticosteroids, below); inhaled CS may cause cough, hoarseness and fungal infection (Candida) in the oropharynx. Ensure that patient rinses mouth after therapy and add spacer to MDI to ↓ risk

Beclomethasone [Beclovent, Vanceril]	MDI: 2 puffs tid, qid of 42 μg (max 20 puffs/d); 2 puffs of 84 μg bid (max 10 puffs/d)
Budesonide [Pulmicort Respules]	DPI: 1 - 4 inh bid of 200 μgNeb: 0.25 - 0.50 mg/2 ml unit dose [1st approved neb CS]
Dexamethasone [Decadron]	MDI: 3 puffs of 84 μg tid, qid (1st MDI steroid in USA; NOT used often since advent of newer steroid agents)
Flunisolide [Aerobid]	MDI: 2 - 4 puffs bid (250 μg/puff)
Fluticasone [Flovent, Flonase]	MDI: 2 - 4 puffs bid of 44, 110 or 220 μg/puff DPI: 1 - 2 inh bid of 50, 100 or 250 μg/inh (also comes combined with Serevent in DPI called Advair)
Triamcinolone [Azmacort]	MDI: 2 puffs tid, qid or 4 puffs bid (of 100 μg/puff), max 16 puffs/d; (comes with built-in spacer)

Systemic corticosteroids:

AE: long-term use: immunosuppression, osteoporosis, fluid retention, hypo-thalamo-pituitary-adrenal suppression, skin bruising, cataract, myopathy of skeletal muscle, glaucoma, Cushing's syndrome (obesity, moon face, buffalo hump in upper back), growth inhibition in children?; **short-term use:** mood changes (euphoria, delirium), hyperglycemia, stomach upset, insomnia, agitation, ↑ appetite

Betamethasone ([Celestone)	Ind: to hasten fetal lung maturity, inflammatory disease
Cortisone [Cortone]	Ind: adrenal insufficiency, inflammatory disease
Dexamethasone [Decadron]	Ind: to hasten fetal lung maturity, cerebral edema, BPD, croup, anaphylaxis
Hydrocortisone [Cortef, A-hydrocort, Solu-Cortef]	Ind: adrenal insufficiency, inflammatory disease (PO, IM, IV)

Methylprednisolone [Medrol, Solu-Medrol]	Ind: acute severe asthma, anaphylaxis, lupus nephritis, spinal cord injury; [PO, IM, IV]
Prednisolone [Prelone]	Ind: acute severe asthma; dose: 5 - 60 mg PO/IV/IM qid; (in children: 1 - 2 mg/kg/d)
Prednisone [Deltasone]	Ind: asthma exacerbations; dose: 5 - 60 mg PO qid (tab: 1, 5, 10, 20, 50 mg or sol 5 mg/5 ml)
Triamcinolone [Aristocort, Kenalog]	Ind: inflammatory disease, dose: 4 - 48 mg/d PO/IM qid

19.3 Asthma/COPD Combinations

Fluticasone + salmeterol [Advair diskus]	DPI: 1 puff bid
Albuterol + ipratropium [Combivent]	MDI: 2 puffs qid
Albuterol + ipratropium [DuoNeb]	Neb: 3 mg albuterol + 0.5 mg ipratropium premixed/3 ml vial

19.4 Non-Steroidal Antiasthmatic Agents

Leukotriene modifiers:
MA: interrupt synthesis of leukotrienes, which contribute to airflow obstruction in asthma patients
Leukotriene receptor blockers: Singulair and Accolate
Leukotriene synthesis inhibitor: Zyflo
Ind: NOT for acute therapy; may be used as alternative to low-dose inhaled steroids or cromones for prophylaxis in mild persistent asthma
AE: headache, dizziness, dyspepsia (indigestion); patients should have liver function monitored

Montelukast [Singulair]	Adults and children ≥ 15 years: 10 mg tab/d; 6 - 14 years: 5 mg tab/d; 2- 5 years: 4 mg tab/d
Zafirlukast [Accolate]	20 mg tab bid; 5 - 11 years: 10 mg tab bid
Zileuton [Zyflo]	600 mg tab qid > 12 years

Cromones: (aka mast-cell stabilizers)
MA: prevent release of inflammatory mediators from mast cells by inhibiting Ca influx into mast cell
Ind: prophylaxis for mild-moderate allergic asthma, exercise-induced asthma; other uses: allergic rhinitis (Nasalcrom), allergic conjunctivitis [Opticrom], mastocytosis [Gastrocrom]

| Cromolyn [Intal] | MDI: 2 - 4 puffs qid; Neb: 20 mg/2 ml vial (may mix with albuterol) |
| Nedocromil [Tilade] | MDI: 2 puffs bid, qid |

19.5 Mucolytic Agents

Acetylcysteine (Mucomyst)

MA	Thins out thick secretions by disrupting disulfide bonds in mucus $\Rightarrow \downarrow$ viscosity. Must refrigerate after opening, discard after 72h or if discolored
Ind	To treat thick secretions: CF, chronic bronchitis. Antidote (PO, diluted in juice) for acetaminophen (Tylenol) OD to $\downarrow$ its toxic effects on liver
Dose	Neb: 3 - 5 ml of 20% or 6 - 10 ml of 10% sol tid, qid ETT, TT instillation: 1 - 2 ml of either sol q1 - q4 h
AE	Bronchospasm (predose or use with bronchodilator), mucus plug secondary to overmobilization of secretions, vomiting, bad smell (rotten eggs), rhinorrhea, stomatitis

Dornase alfa (Pulmozyme)

MA	Thins out thick secretions by breaking down DNA of mucus $\Rightarrow \downarrow$ viscosity and adhesiveness, which helps mobilize secretions
Ind	CF patients with thick secretions
Dose	Neb: 2.5 mg in 2.5 ml sol qd - bid
AE	Voice alteration, rash, chest pain, conjunctivitis

19.6 Inhaled Antimicrobial Agents

Pentamidine (NebuPent)

MA	**Antiprotozoal**: inhibits DNA, RNA, phospholipids and protein synthesis
Ind	Therapy and prophylaxis of *Pneumocystis carinii* which causes *Pneumocystis carinii* pneumonia (PCP). PCP is often seen in AIDS patients
Dose	300 mg powder vial diluted in 6 ml sterile H_2O q4 weeks via approved neb with 1-way insp valve and expir filter to ↓ exposure (e.g. Respigard II nebulizer)
AE	Give in -ve pressure room [at least 6 air changes/h] or isolation booth; pregnant or breast-feeding mothers should avoid exposure; may cause bronchospasm to patient (pretreat with β_2 agonist); exposure to caregiver: bronchospasm, conjunctivitis, risk of TB (use gloves, mask, eyewear)

Ribavirin (Virazole)

MA	**Antiviral**: (virostatic, not virucidal) may disrupt DNA synthesis
Ind	For patients who have or are at high risk for, severe RSV infection (pneumonia, bronchiolitis). NOT used often, due to lack of objective data, expensive, hazards + introduction of new prophylactic drugs for RSV (RSV-IGIV [RespiGam and Palivizumab [Synagys])
Dose	6 g/300 ml sterile H_2O by SPAG neb for 12 - 18 h/d for 3 - 7 days
AE	Teratogenic (embryocidal)/carcinogenic (pregnant patients and staff should avoid it); conjunctivitis, headache, rash, dizziness, pharyngitis

Tobramycin (TOBI)

MA	**Antibiotic** for Gram+ve and Gram-ve organisms; bacteriocidal
Ind	Chronic infections with *P. aeruginosa* in CF patients
Dose	> 6 years: neb: 300 mg/5 ml ampule q12 h, 28 d on 28 d off
AE	Voice alteration, tinnitus (subjective ringing noise in ears)

Zanamivir (Relenza)

MA	**Antiviral**: inhibits neuraminidase
Ind	Influenza: acute therapy (note that best therapy against flu is vaccination)
Dose	DPI: > 12 years, 2 inh bid x 5 d
AE	Bronchospasm (discontinue drug if it occurs), diarrhea, nausea, dizziness

19.7 Surfactants

Ind: premature infants with RDS
Prevention: infant at high risk for RDS (LBW: < 1.3 kg, < 32 weeks, lecithin to sphingomyelin (L:S) ratio < 2:1 and absence of phosphatidylglycerol (PG)
Rescue therapy: grunting, nasal flare, retractions, cyanosis, ↑ O_2 requirement, 'ground-glass' CXR appearance. Instilled directly into trachea through ETT Administration method varies on the type used. Patient repositioning is required to ensure homogeneous distribution

Beractant (Survanta): 4 ml/kg given in 4 divided doses in 4 positions by direct side-port ETT instillation or through a 5-F catheter placed in ETT

Calfactant (Infasurf): 3 ml/kg by direct side-port ETT delivery or through a catheter in 2 divided doses of 1.5 ml/kg

Colfosceril (Exosurf): 5 ml/kg reconstituted in 2 doses and instilled by direct side-port ETT. Give in burst and turn infant to right side for 30 s and then left for 30 s

Poractant (Curosurf): 2.5 ml/kg directly through catheter placed in ETT in 2 half doses in 2 positions

BIBLIOGRAPHY

Colbert BJ, Mason BJ: Integrated Cardiopulmonary Pharmacology, Prentice Hall, 2001.

Rau J: Respiratory Care Pharmacology, 6th ed. Mosby 2002.

Russ A: Drug Pocket: Clinical Reference Guide, 2nd ed. Börm Bruckmeier Publishing, 2003.

20. Medical Gas Therapy

20.1 Oxygen Therapy

Indications
- Documented hypoxemia
  - In adults, children and infants > 28 days old, hypoxemia exists when $PaO_2 < 60$ mmHg or $SaO_2 < 90\%$ on room air
  - In infants ≤ 28 days old, hypoxemia exists when $PaO_2 < 50$ mmHg and $SaO_2 < 88\%$
- Emergency situations such as:
  - Severe respiratory distress
  - Shock
  - Cardiopulmonary arrest/MI
  - Carbon monoxide poisoning
  - Severe trauma
- Suspected hypoxemia
- Excessive work of breathing
- Excessive myocardial work

AARC Clinical Practice Guideline

Oxygen therapy for adults in the acute care facility	

Indications	• Documented hypoxemia
	  ○ $PaO_2 < 60$ mmHg or
	    $SaO_2 < 90\%$
	  ○ Also, suspected hypoxemia in acute care situations
	  ○ Acute MI
	  ○ Severe trauma
	• Short-term therapy (e.g. postoperative)

Contraindications	• None

Monitoring of patient	○ Clinical assessment
	○ PaO_2 or SaO_2 with initiation of therapy or within:
	  – 12 hours on $FIO_2 < 0.40$
	  – 8 hours on $FIO_2 > 0.40$
	  – 72 hours in acute MI, 2 hours in COPD

Precautions/possible complications	• Ventilatory depression:
	  ◦ In patients with elevated $PaCO_2$ and $PaO_2 > 60$ mmHg
	• With $FIO_2 > 0.50$
	  ◦ Absorption atelectasis
	  ◦ Oxygen toxicity
	  ◦ ↓ Ciliary function
	  ◦ ↓ Leukocyte function
	• Caution in patients with:
	  ◦ Paraquat poisoning
	  ◦ Receiving bleomycin
	• Fire hazard
	• Bacterial contamination (humidification systems)
	• During laser bronchoscopy, minimal levels of O_2 should be used to avoid intratracheal ignition
	• Equipment:
	  ◦ All equipment checked at least once/day
	  ◦ More frequent when:
	    - Clinically unstable
	    - $FIO_2 > 0.50$
	    - Heated gas mixture
	    - Artificial airways
	• Blending gas systems

Frequency	• Continuous, unless need only with specific situation (e.g. exercise, sleep)

From AARC Clinical Practice Guideline: Oxygen Therapy in the Acute Care Facility, Respir Care 2002; 47: 717-720.

20.1.1 Hypoxemia versus Hypoxia

• Hypoxemia: ↓ amount of O_2 in the blood (↓ PaO_2, ↓ SaO_2 and/or ↓ CaO_2)
• Hypoxia: ↓ amount of O_2 at tissue level
• Anoxia: absent tissue oxygen

Effectiveness of oxygen therapy in different forms of hypoxia

Hypoxemic hypoxia	
Causes and examples	• ↓ inspired O_2 tension due to high altitude (↓ Pb) or patient not receiving prescribed O_2 • Alveolar hypoventilation: drug overdose, NM weakness, OSA • V/Q mismatch: COPD, asthma, diffuse lung disease • R – L shunt: pulmonary edema, ARDS, pneumonia, atelectasis
Response to O_2	Mostly good, except in R – L shunt
Anemic hypoxia	
Mechanism	Hypoxia due to ↓ O_2 carrying capacity of the blood
Examples	Severe anemia, carbon monoxide poisoning, Hb disease, severe blood loss
Response to O_2	None; possibly in borderline situations
Circulatory (stagnant or hypoperfusion) hypoxia	
Mechanism	Hypoxia due to ↓ blood flow in the body
Examples	MI, CHF, shock, hypovolemia
Response to O_2	Poor
Histotoxic hypoxia	
Mechanism	Hypoxia due to inability of cells to use O_2
Examples	Cyanide poisoning (cellular respiration inhibited)
Response to O_2	Poor

20.1.2 Hazards of oxygen therapy

Absorption atelectasis:
• Administering high FIO_2 ⇒ washes out N_2 from alveoli
  (N_2 is normally ~ 80% in alveoli)
• Oxygen is removed from alveoli faster than it can be replaced by normal ventilation
  which ⇒ ↓ alveolar size ⇒ alveolar collapse/atelectasis

Retinopathy of prematurity:
- Vascular proliferation disease of retina
- High PaO_2 causes vasoconstriction of blood vessels behind retina $\Rightarrow \downarrow$ blood flow
  - Developing vessels may permanently constrict, which $\Rightarrow$ necrosis (vaso-obliteration)
  - New vessels form to oxygenate the eye, which may $\Rightarrow$ retinal clouding and scarring
  - Scar tissue from the hemorrhage shrinks $\Rightarrow$ retinal detachment and blindness
- $\uparrow$ **risk with:**
  - Infant < 33 weeks of age and < 1.5 kg weight
  - $\uparrow$ Exposure to O_2 with PaO_2 > 80 - 100 mmHg
  - Retinal vessel immaturity.

Treatment/prevention:
  - Maintain PaO_2 at 50 - 80 mmHg
  - $\downarrow$ Exposure time to high FIO_2
  - Laser surgery for glaucoma

Oxygen toxicity:
- Use of high O_2% (> 50 - 60%) for prolonged periods (> 2 - 3 days?) may $\Rightarrow$ destruction of alveolar type I cells and their replacement with type II cells. Edema and destruction/necrosis of endothelial cells follows $\Rightarrow$ hyaline membrane disease
- In the newborn, these pathologic changes are referred to as BPD
- $\downarrow$ Risk of oxygen toxicity by using PEEP when FIO_2 is ≥ 0.50

Oxygen-induced hypoventilation:
- Rare: found in small % of patients with CO_2 retention. These patients are breathing as a result of stimulation of aortic and carotid chemoreceptors secondary to severe hypoxia
- When high levels of oxygen are given, $\uparrow PaO_2$ apparently eliminates the drive to breathe $\Rightarrow$ hypoventilation/apnea

Ductus arteriosus (DA) closure/constriction:
- $\uparrow PaO_2$ contributes to closure/constriction of DA post-birth
- DA closure is a concern in infants with heart defects that require DA to be open (DA-dependent heart defects)

20.1.3 Oxygen delivery devices

Nasal cannula (NC)	Delivers **24 – 44%** O_2 at 1 – 6 L/min flow rate (each ↑ 1 L/min ~ ↑ 4% O_2). Appropriate device for **COPD** patient. Generally, flows ≤ 4 L/min do not need to be humidified. **Infants:** limit max flow to ≤ 2 L/min (NC is usually taped to face in these patients)	**Flow rate** 1 L/min 2 L/min 3 L/min 4 L/min 5 L/min 6 L/min	O_2% 24% 28% 32% 36% 40% 44%
Simple O_2 mask	Delivers: **35 – 55%** O_2 at flows of 5 – 8 L/min. Must use flows ≥ 5 L/min to ensure flushing of CO_2 out of mask. **Not** tolerated by many patients		
Venturi mask	aka air-entrainment mask (AEM). Delivers specific FIO_2 up to 0.50 (**24 – 50%** O_2). Recommended for **COPD** patients as an initial O_2 device (suspected hypoxic drive or unsure). Uses a series of exact concentration adaptors that are attached to a mask to determine exact FIO_2 by mixing entrained air and pure oxygen	2 L/min 3 L/min 4 L/min 6 L/min 8 L/min 10 L/min 12 L/min	24% 28% 32% 35% 40% 45% 50%
Non-rebreathing mask (NRM)	Delivers **90 – 100%** O_2 at 10 – 15 L/min flow with perfect conditions (e.g. tight seal, 3 one-way valves instead of 2), which is rare. Therefore, delivered O_2 is probably **70 – 80%** at best. **Must** be run with sufficient flow to prevent bag collapse on inspiration. Used for **emergencies**: CHF, PTX, carbon monoxide poisoning and burns + delivery of He-O_2 gas mixtures. It has a one-way valve between the bag and mask, which prevents exhaled gas from entering the bag and a one-way valve at the exhalation side port, which prevents inspiration from room air.		

NOTE: *Some inspiration from room air does occur due to inability to provide airtight seal and missing of 3rd one-way exhalation side port valve (designed for safety reasons in case O_2 source runs out undetected, thereby allowing patient to at least draw in room air).*

Partial rebreathing mask	**Not** used often. Same as nonrebreathing mask except that the flap valve between reservoir bag and mask is removed. Delivers **40 - 70%** O_2 at liter flow (10 - 15L/min) that keeps the bag $^2/_3$ full on inspiration to prevent CO_2 rebreathing.

Newborn/pediatric O_2- Devices

Oxygen (head) hood	Transparent plastic hood that fits around infant's/newborn's head. Humidified O_2 is delivered to hood by corrugated tubing attached to either air-entrainment heated nebulizer (32 - 34 °C) or blender with heated humidifier. **Minimum** flow of > 7 L/min should be used to prevent CO_2 buildup. FIO_2 must be continuously monitored with O_2 analyzer near patient's head. This device can also be used inside incubators.
Oxygen (mist) tent	Delivers **40 - 50%** O_2 at best (or room air) at flows > 10 - 15 L/min coming from large volume nebulizer. Used for croup, bronchiolitis and pneumonia patients. Transparent canopy must be tucked into mattress to prevent loss of O_2.
Incubator (closed)	Used for controlling temperature, O_2, humidity. Provides **40 - 50%** O_2 at flows 8 - 15 L/min. May provide up to 100% O_2 on some models. O_2 can also be provided via O_2 hood placed inside the incubator

NOTE: *Radiant warmer is an open incubator used for providing neutral thermal environment.*

Aerosol devices used for O_2- delivery

Air entrainment nebulizer	aka large volume nebulizer (LVN). Delivers high humidity with specific FIO_2 which is adjusted by manipulating air entrainment ports. Must ensure adequate flow (seeing mist on inspiration usually indicates adequate flow). May be heated by placing on heating device. Used for delivering humidified O_2 (via corrugated tubing) to aerosol mask, tracheostomy collar, T-piece or face tent.

T-piece	Small T-shaped adaptor that fits on ETT on one end; on the other end, corrugated tubing, which delivers humidified O_2 from air entrainment nebulizer, is attached. Used for T-piece weaning from mechanical ventilation. Clinician should ensure that on inspiration, mist is seen coming out of reservoir tubing (~ 15 cm long) to ensure adequate flow to patient.
Aerosol mask, tracheostomy collar, face tent	Used for delivering humidified O_2 coming from air entrainment nebulizer via corrugated tubing. **Aerosol mask:** often used for delivering humidified O_2 post-extubation. A small volume medication delivery nebulizer can be attached to this mask (sometimes comes pre-packaged) for patients who are unable to use hand-held nebulizer. **Tracheostomy collar** or trach mask is commonly used for delivering O_2 to patients with TT in place. **Face tent** is rarely used. It may be of temporary benefit in patients with facial burns or disfigurement due to accidents (e.g. car crash).

Home/long-term O_2 - devices

Trans-tracheal O_2 catheter	No. 8 or 9 French catheter is inserted surgically between 2nd and 3rd tracheal rings and extends ~ 3 cm above carina. Since O_2 is delivered directly to trachea, O_2 can be ↓ by ~ 50%. Held in place by neck chain (cosmetic appearance). Routine care: site cleaning, lavaging, cleaning with a rod to remove mucus. It should also be replaced every 3 months. Not popular with patients due to require-ment of surgical procedure and the possible complications of having catheter in place: infections, bleeding, mucus obstruction. It may also not be covered by medical insurance plans.
Concentrator	Runs on electricity and is often used in nursing homes or at home. N_2 is extracted from air leaving O_2 for patient delivery, usually via nasal cannula. Maximum delivered flow rate is ~ 5 - 6 L/min. Bubble humidifier, if needed, can be attached to it. Newer units provide 2 connections, but each connection cannot be used for > 3 L/min. Need backup (O_2 tanks) in case of power failure.

Cylinders	Large **'H'** cylinder is often used as a stationary O_2 source, while smaller **'E'** cylinder is used for portable use (transport, trip). Cheap method of delivering O_2 at home, but may be difficult to change and move around for older people. • When full, cylinders are filled to 2200 psi (pounds per square inch). For safety reasons, it is standard practice to replace the tank once it reaches 500 psi	Calculating how long (duration of flow in min) the cylinder will last Equation: **Duration of flow (in min)** $$= \frac{\text{gauge pressure x tank factor}}{\text{Liter flow}}$$ [tank factor: 'H' cylinder 3.14 and 'E' cylinder 0.28]
Liquid O_2 systems	Last longer than cylinders (860.0 of O_2 gas/L of liquid is stored). Large size units are used for hospitals and ventilator units, while small portable size units are used for home care. **Stationary units** at home can provide O_2 for 4 - 12 days at ~ 2 L/min flow. **Smaller portable liquid system units** are light (5 - 13 lb or ~ 2.5 - 7.5 kg) and can easily be refilled from a main stationary liquid reservoir, but this should be done carefully as there is a risk of frostbite/skin damage because it is very cold. Portable liquid systems contain 0.5 - 1.5 L of liquid O_2 which can last up to 24 hours at low flow rates (e.g. 1 L/min). These systems are usually the most expensive delivery system for home use.	

Other O_2 - delivery devices

Bag mask ventilator (BMV)	(Resuscitator bag): Self inflating, rugby ball shaped device with O_2 reservoir that is mostly used for emergency situations to deliver ~ 100% O_2 (e.g. CPR or patient transport at short distance; connected to 'E' tank). Flow of oxygen must be kept high enough (15 L/min) to keep the bag from deflating substantially. **Placement:** can be placed over patient's face, covering the mouth and nose or the mask is removed and the standard 15/22 mm inside/outside diameter fitting is connected to patient's artificial airway.

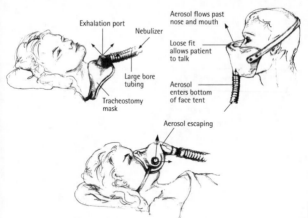

Exhalation port

Nebulizer

Large bore tubing

Tracheostomy mask

Aerosol flows past nose and mouth

Loose fit allows patient to talk

Aerosol enters bottom of face tent

Aerosol escaping

Fig. 32 Illustrating aerosol mask, face tent, T-piece and tracheostomy mask (collar) connected to air entrainment nebulizer, which can be set up to provide humidified oxygen from cylinder or wall oxygen supply.

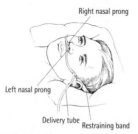

Right nasal prong

Left nasal prong

Delivery tube   Restraining band

Fig. 33 Nasal cannula

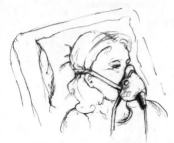

Fig. 34 Simple oxygen mask

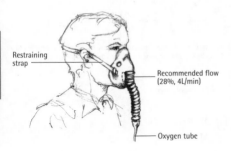

Restraining
strap

Recommended flow
(28%, 4L/min)

Oxygen tube

Fig. 35 Venturi or air entrainment mask (AEM)

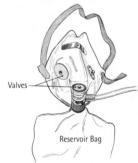

Valves

Reservoir Bag

Fig. 36 Nonrebreathing mask

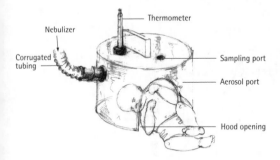

Thermometer

Nebulizer

Corrugated tubing

Sampling port

Aerosol port

Hood opening

Fig. 37 Typical infant oxygen hood

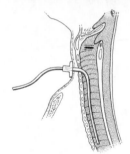

Fig. 38 Transtracheal O_2 catheter in place

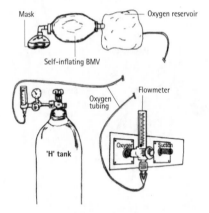

Fig. 39 Shows resuscitator (bag-mask valve unit) and oxygen source to which it can be attached: large 'H' oxygen tank and wall oxygen source mostly found in hospitals

20.2 Hyperbaric Oxygen Therapy

Description

- Hyperbaric oxygen therapy (HBO) is the administration of O_2 at pressures greater than atmospheric. HBO increases the amount of O_2 in the blood and tissues
- At 1 atmosphere (760 mmHg) $PaO_2 \approx 100$ mmHg on room air, which = dissolved O_2 of only ~ 0.3 ml/dl
- At 3 atmosphere (2280 mmHg [760 mmHg x 3]) $PaO_2 \sim 1800$ at 100% O_2 and dissolved O_2 in plasma is ~ 6 ml/dl

Indications and probable mechanism of HBO

- Carbon monoxide poisoning:
  - Usually normal O_2 can be achieved using 100% O_2 with nonrebreather mask
  - HBO is usually considered when COHb is > 30 - 40% and hyperbaric facility is available
  - HBO forces carbon monoxide off the hemoglobin molecule
- Infections
  - Gas gangrene (Clostridial myonecrosis)
  - Refractory osteomyelitis
  - HBO inactivates the toxin
- Air bubble disease
  - Gas embolism
  - Decompression sickness
  - HBO increases pressures which decrease bubble size
- Cyanide poisoning
- Thermal injury (burns)
  - HBO reduces edema and infection and accelerates wound healing

Hazards and complications of HBO

- Barotrauma (PTX)
  - Due to increased pressures
- Tympanic membrane rupture
  - Due to occluded Eustachian tubes
- Other complications:
  - O_2 toxicity, fire, claustrophobia

Administration

HBO can be administered in a single (monoplace) chamber or multiplace chamber

Using ventilators in a chamber

- Ventilator should be small, portable, able to work on an internal battery for many hours and the pressures it delivers to the patient should not be affected by changing pressures in the chamber
- It is recommended that the ETT cuff be filled with H_2O to avoid continual adjustment of cuff valve during chamber compression and decompression. Without H_2O, ETT cuff is compressed due to increased ambient pressure, which leads to loss of seal

20.3 Helium – Oxygen (He-O_2) Therapy

Description

- Since helium has a much lower density than O_2, it may be of value in the treatment of airway obstruction. It decreases airway resistance by helping the gas mixture move through the airways. It enhances delivery of O_2 and medicated aerosol. Helium is also inert and has no medicinal value if used by itself
- He-O_2 mixtures are provided in 2 forms:

1. 80 – 20 mixture: 80% He, 20% O_2

2. 70 – 30 mixture: 70% He, 30% O_2; this mixture is used when additional O_2 is needed to correct hypoxemia resulting from airway obstruction

Possible indications

1. Upper airway obstruction
2. Status asthmaticus
3. Refractory croup

Administration

1. Tight-fitting nonrebreathing mask. Note that small volume medication nebulizer can be connected via a 'Y' connector to the nonrebreather mask so that He-O_2 mixture and bronchodilators can be delivered at the same time
2. ETT (cuffed) if intubated

Side effects

Benign: temporary distortion of voice

Things to consider

- Because of difference in gas density, an O_2 flowmeter will not provide an accurate reading of the actual flow rate used. The conversion factor used to correct this problem is: 1.6 for the 70/30 He-O_2 mixture and 1.8 for the 80/20 He-O_2 mixture

- Therefore, correct flow used = 1.6 x flow used (for 70/30 He-O_2 mixture) and 1.8 x flow used (for 80/20 He-O_2 mixture)
- Example: if the flowmeter reads 12 L/min, about 21 - 22 L/min would be the actual flow for the 80/20 He-O_2 mixture

20.4 Nitric Oxide (NO) Therapy

Description
- NO is an endothelial-derived relaxing factor. When it is inhaled, it causes selective pulmonary vasodilation (NO = pulmonary vasodilator)
- Pulmonary vasodilation $\Rightarrow$ ↓ pulmonary vascular resistance (PVR) $\Rightarrow$ ↑ oxygenation (without causing systemic hypotension) due to dilation of pulmonary vessels in better ventilated lung areas

Indications
- PPHN
- Postoperatively in patients who develop PH due to surgical repair of congenital heart disease
- Possibly: severe hypoxemia due to IRDS, pneumonia, MAS, sepsis

Delivery systems
- Inhaled NO can be delivered either through ETT (intubated patients) connected to ventilator breathing circuit or the same delivery systems can be adapted to deliver NO via nasal cannula
- FDA approved inhaled NO device: iNOvent Delivery Systems (by Ohmeda)

Recommended dose
$\geq$ 20 ppm with oxygen

Potential adverse effects
- **Methemoglobinemia:** due to overdose
  - It is important to scavenge NO if using $\geq$ 80 ppm
  - Monitor metHb levels (acceptable level < 5%)
- **Lung injury:** due to nitrogen dioxide (NO_2)
  - NO converts quickly to NO_2 in the presence of oxygen
  - NO_2 must be continuously monitored in the inhaled NO circuit

BIBLIOGRAPHY

Ward JJ: Medical Gas Therapy. In, Burton GG, Hodgkin JE, Ward JJ et al (eds): Respiratory Care: A Guide to Clinical Practice, 4th ed. LWW, 1997.

Saposnick AB, Hess DR: Oxygen Therapy. In, Hess DR et al (eds): Respiratory Care: Principles and Practice, WB Saunders, 2002.

Heuer AJ, Scanlan CL: Medical Gas Therapy. In, Wilkins RL, Stoller JK, Scanlan CL (eds): Egan's Fundamentals of Respiratory Care, 8th ed. Elsevier Science Limited, 2003.

21. Ventilator Management

21.1 Indications for Mechanical Ventilation

21.1.1 Respiratory failure

Respiratory failure (RF) is not a disease, but is the end result of any abnormality which interferes with any part of the respiratory system: respiratory center (medulla), respiratory muscles, chest wall, lungs, airways and alveoli. RF is divided into ventilatory 'pump' failure and oxygenation 'lung' failure.

21.1.2 Ventilatory failure

Definition
Inadequate CO_2 elimination secondary to hypoventilation: $\downarrow V_A = \uparrow PaCO_2$.
Also known as hypercapnic respiratory failure

Etiology
Some examples:

CNS depression
($\downarrow$ respiratory drive); CVA, trauma, drug OD, lesions

Chest wall
Kyphoscoliosis, PTX, obesity, flail chest

Neuromuscular
GBS, MG, ALS, phrenic nerve injury, hypo-K, Mg, PO_4

Lungs/airways
Severe asthma, COPD, ARDS, upper airway obstruction

Diagnosis
Likely ABGs

- $\uparrow$ **$PaCO_2$** > 50 - 55 mmHg and rising or acute $\uparrow$ by > 5 - 10 mmHg above baseline in chronic hypercapnia (COPD)
- $\downarrow$ **PaO_2** secondary to $\uparrow PaCO_2$
- **Normal P(A – a)O2** gradient

21.1.3 Oxygenation failure

Definition

Inadequate gas exchange at A-C membrane
It is also known as hypoxemic respiratory failure

Etiology

Some examples:

- **Ventilation–perfusion (V/Q mismatch):** most common cause of hypoxemia (COPD, asthma, atelectasis); $\uparrow FIO_2 \Rightarrow \uparrow PaO_2$
- **Shunt:** ARDS, severe pneumonia, pulmonary edema; $\uparrow FIO_2 \neq \uparrow PaO_2$
- **Hypoventilation:** secondary to hypercapnic RF ($\uparrow PaCO_2 \Rightarrow \downarrow PaO_2$)
- **Diffusion impairment:** rare
- **Decreased inspired oxygen ($\downarrow PIO_2$):**
  rare cause; high altitude ($\downarrow PB$) or smoke inhalation

Diagnosis

- $\downarrow PaO_2 < 60$ mmHg on $FIO_2 > 0.60$
- **Normal or $\downarrow PaCO_2$** ($\uparrow$ in hypoventilation)
- **$\uparrow P(A - a)O_2$ gradient** (normal in hypoventilation)

21.1.4 Other indications

- Apnea
- Major thoracic or abdominal surgery
- Closed head trauma: temporary hyperventilation (lowering of $PaCO_2$ to ~ 25 - 30 mmHg) to $\downarrow$ intracranial pressure (ICP).

NOTE: Mechanical ventilation does not cure the underlying disorder; it only supports the respiratory system until the cause is corrected.

Summary: Parameters that may indicate the need for ventilatory support

Parameter	Normal range	MV indicated
Mechanics		
Respiratory rate (RR) - breaths/min	12 - 20	≥ 35
Vital capacity (V_C) - ml/kg	60 - 75	< 10 - 15
Maximum inspiratory pressure (MIP) - cmH_2O	70 - 100	< 25
Maximum voluntary ventilation (MVV) - L/min	120 - 180	< 20 or $\leq 2 \times V_E$

Rapid shallow breathing index; ratio of RR to V_T in L - (RR/V_T)		> 100
Ventilation		
$PaCO_2$ - mmHg	35 - 45	> 55 and rising
pH	7.35 - 7.45	< 7.25
Tidal volume (V_T) - ml/kg ideal body weight	5 - 8	< 3
Minute ventilation (V_E) - L/min	5 - 8	> 12 - 15
Dead space ventilation (V_D/V_T)	25 - 40%	> 60%
Oxygenation		
PaO_2 - mmHg	75 - 100 (room air)	< 60 on FIO_2 > 0.6
A - a gradient ($PAO_2 - PaO_2$)	5 - 20 (air) < 65 (100% O_2)	> 350 on 100% O_2
PaO_2/FIO_2	350 - 450	< 200
PaO_2/PAO_2	0.75 - 0.95	< 0.15
Qs/Qt (shunt %)	≤ 5	> 20 - 30

21.2 Complications of Mechanical Ventilation

NOTE: Assisted ventilation is often life saving, but can also cause complications which the clinician should be familiar with, in order to minimize them.

21.2.1 Potential complications of positive pressure ventilation (PPV)

Barotrauma/volutrauma
- Excessive persistent airway pressure and excessive inflating volumes may
  $\Rightarrow$ alveolar stretch injury which leads to PTX or other pulmonary air leaks such as pulmonary interstitial emphysema (PIE)
- ↑ **risk:**
(1) P_{plat} > 30 cmH$_2$O
(2) PIP > 50 cmH$_2$O
(3) V_T > 12 - 15 ml/kg

(4) PEEP > 10 - 15 cmH$_2$O
- **PIP:** less reliable indicator than P$_{plat}$ because it reflects factors not influencing P$_{alv}$ (↑ R$_{aw}$: small ETT, secretions, bronchospasm) and mostly dissipates in large airways
- **P$_{plat}$ ≈ P$_{alv}$** = more useful than PIP, but PIP is also good to follow as a trending indicator of barotrauma

Decreased cardiac output (↓ CO)
- PPV ⇒ ↑ intrathoracic pressure which ⇒ compressed heart and vena cavas ⇒ ↓ venous return to right heart (↓ RV filling) = ↓ CO

Decreased blood pressure (↓ BP)
- **Hypotension** usually occurs secondary to ↓ CO
- ↑ Risk: hypovolemia and ↓ cardiac reserve

Decreased urinary output (↓ UO)
- ↓ CO ⇒ ↓ renal blood flow and filtration pressures ⇒ ↓ UO
- Diuretics as needed

Increased intracranial pressure (↑ ICP)
- Compressed vena cavas ⇒ blood pools in head = ↑ ICP
- Negligible with PEEP < 10 cmH$_2$O and patients without head injury

NOTE: *Degree of negative effect depends on level of PPV (↑ if PEEP used, especially > 10 cmH$_2$O) and amount of pressure transmitted to pulmonary vasculature (↓ with ↓ C$_L$). Negative hemodynamic effects of PPV are often minimized or corrected with fluids ± inotropes.*

Oxygen toxicity
- FIO$_2$ > 0.5 - 0.6 for > 48 - 72 hours (?) may be toxic to lung tissue (ARDS-like complication)
- ↓ FIO$_2$ to < 0.5 ASAP

Ventilator–associated pneumonia (VAP)
- Usually secondary to aspiration of contaminated oral secretions.
  Diagnosis: fever > 38°C, ↑ WBC, ↓ PaO$_2$, purulent secretion, CXR = new/progressive infiltrates, (+) ET aspiration/brush culture
- ↓ Risk: elevate HOB > 30°, good oral care, sterile suction, use HME if not contraindicated and do not change ventilator circuit often (q7 - 14 days or prn)

Airway complications
- **During intubation:** misplaced ETT into esophagus or main bronchus; upper airway trauma (broken teeth, cuts)

- **While intubated:** laryngeal web, edema, stenosis or vocal cords ulcer; cuff pressure > 25 - 35 cmH$_2$O > 18 - 25 mmHg) = ↑ risk for tracheal stenosis or TE fistula; cuff rupture or herniation; pilot tube cut; accidental extubation

Ventilator problems

- Ventilator malfunction, oxygen failure, electrical failure, leaks or disconnections in the circuit
- Each mechanically ventilated patient should have AMBU (resuscitation bag) at their bedside in case of emergency need for bag ventilation

Auto-PEEP

Definition

Unintentional PEEP during MV. It occurs when inspiration starts prior to end of expiration (inadequate Te) ⇒ air trapping

If severe

= ↑ barotrauma risk + ↑ WOB as patient has to inspire through both auto-PEEP and sensitivity to trigger a breath

Causes

Fast RR, high V$_E$, airflow obstruction and ↑ R$_{aw}$

Measure

By occluding exhalation valve or pressing expiratory hold button (found on many ventilators) at the end of exhalation (autoPEEP = totPEEP - setPEEP)

Treatment

↑ Te (↑ RR, ↑ FR, = ↓ Ti); sedation

21.3 Selecting Initial Ventilator Settings

Tidal volume (V$_T$)

- Set initially at **7 - 10 ml/kg IBW** and adjust so that P$_{plat}$ ≤ 30 cmH$_2$O
- V$_T$ > 12 - 15 ml/kg ⇒ ↑ risk for barotrauma. (Normal spont V$_T$ ≈ 5 - 8 ml/kg)
- For ARDS/COPD patients: 5 - 6 ml/kg is normally used

Respiratory rate (RR)

- Set initially at **10 - 14 breaths/min**
- RR ≤ 8 breaths/min is often used for COPD/airway obstruction to ↑ expiratory time (Te) which ⇒ ↓ air trapping
- RR ≥ 16 breaths/min is commonly used for restrictive lung disorders (↓ C$_L$) which require small V$_T$ to prevent barotrauma

Fraction of inspired oxygen (FIO₂)

- Set initially at **0.7 – 1.0** if no baseline ABG initially. ↓ ASAP to < 0.5 (to accomplish this, use PEEP if necessary)
- $FIO_2 > 0.5 - 0.6$ for > 48 - 72 hours ⇒ O_2 toxicity?

PEEP/CPAP

- **PEEP** stands for Positive End-Expiratory Pressure, **PEEP** = applying (+ve) pressure > atmospheric at end expiration
- **CPAP** stands for Constant Positive Airway Pressure. **CPAP** = PEEP applied to spontaneous breaths
- Set at: **zero initially;** for refractory hypoxemia (PaO_2 < 60 mmHg on FIO_2 > 0.5 - 0.6) start at 5 cmH₂O
- PEEP and CPAP are NOT true modes, but adjuncts or maneuvers designed to improve oxygenation and not provide ventilation. PEEP is used as an adjunct to other modes, while CPAP is mainly used for weaning (patient breathes spontaneously at PEEP)
- **Physiology:** PEEP/CPAP prevent alveolar collapse and recruit collapsed alveoli (↓ atelectasis), ↑ FRC = ↑ C_L = ↓ V/Q mismatch ⇒ ↑ oxygenation
- **Caution:** unilateral lung disease, COPD, PTX, ↑ ICP, hypotension and P_{plat} > 30 cmH₂O usually contraindicate PEEP. Negative effects of PPV ↑ with PEEP: < 10 cmH₂O is usually insignificant, but > 10 cmH₂O usually requires PA catheter to monitor heart function

Sensitivity

- Sensitivity = inspiratory effort that triggers ventilator breath
- **Pressure trigger** set at - **1 to - 2 cmH₂O** < baseline pressure
- **Flow trigger 1 – 3 L/min** < baseline is recommended
- **If set too low** (- 3 cmH₂O) = patient works harder to trigger ⇒ anxiety and ↑ WOB
- **If set too high** (- 0.5 cmH₂O) = possible auto (self) cycling which ⇒ hyperventilat

Flow rate (FR)

- FR (or inspiratory flow) = speed of V_T delivery
- **Initially: 40 - 60 L/min**
- > 60 - 100 L/min is often used for COPD/asthma patients to ↑ Te = ↓ air trapping
- Can be delivered in various patterns such as square or decelerating, but there is no significant advantage between the two

Ti, Te, I:E ratio

- **Inspiratory time (Ti):** of 0.7 - 1.2 seconds is the usual range for adults
- **Expiratory time (Te):** should be $\geq$ 1.5 x Ti in adults
- **Inspiratory to expiratory time ratio (I:E ratio):** should be about 1:3 (meaning that 33% of the respiratory cycle is spent on Ti and 66% on Te)
- I:E ratio of > 1:4 - 1:7 is often used for COPD and asthma patients to promote more complete exhalation

Alarms

Alarms are set in order to get clinician's attention when patient's condition changes. They should not be set at a level so sensitive that they are constantly triggered, which may lead to clinicians ignoring them (this can be dangerous for patient's safety).

General guidelines for setting ventilator alarms:

- **High/low V_E or V_T:** ± 15% above and below set volume
- **High/low PIP:** 15 cmH$_2$O > and 5 - 10 cmH$_2$O < average PIP (start high PIP ↑ 50 cmH$_2$O and adjust)
- **High/low FIO$_2$:** ± 5%
- **Apnea:** ~ 20 seconds
- **High/low RR:** +10 to 15 breaths above set rate and - 5 to 10 breaths below set rate

Humidification

- **Heat moisture exchanger (HME):** start with this unless contraindicated. HME collects patients' exhaled heat/moisture and returns it on next inspiration. HME is also called **artificial nose**
- **Heated humidifier (HH):** standard for neonates + adults with thick secretions, large leaks and need for > 3 HME changes/d. HH is set so that gas temp at airway is 32 - 35°C with high/low temp alarms at 37/30°C

21.4 Ventilatory Modes

Volume-targeted ventilation

- Also known as volumecontrolled [V_C] or volume ventilation [VV]
- Advantage: V_T is constant with lung compliance C_L and/or airway resistance (R_{aw}) changes
- Disadvantages: ↓ C_L and/or ↑R_{aw} results in ↑ PIP $\Rightarrow$ ↑ risk of barotrauma

21.4.1 Assist control (AC)

Description
- The patient receives preset RR of a preset V_T
- In between mandatory breaths, patient can ↑ his or her minute ventilation (V_E) by triggering more breaths of preset V_T. To trigger an additional ventilator breath, the patient must generate a negative inspiratory airway pressure (usually set at -1 to -2 cmH$_2$O below the airway pressure at end expiration)

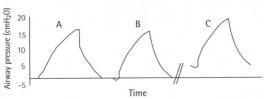

Fig. 40 Assist control

Breath A: mandatory breath, delivered by machine when no inspiratory effort is detected

Breath B: assisted patient-triggered breath; note the negative deflection below end-expiratory pressure

Breath C: assisted breath with positive end-expiratory pressure (PEEP) of 5 cmH$_2$O being used together with AC mode

Indications
- Patients without respiratory effort; e.g. drug OD, CNS injury
- Useful when need to provide full or near full ventilatory support, as in NM weakness or NM blockade
- Usually chosen as initial mode of ventilation

Advantages
- Assures minimum set V_E (V_T x RR)
- Respiratory muscles are rested (minimal WOB)

Disadvantages
- Prolonged use may ⇒ respiratory muscle atrophy
- Possibly alveolar hyperventilation/respiratory alkalosis ± air trapping secondary to:

○ Patient overtriggering the ventilator (e.g. CNS disease, sepsis, pain, fever)
○ Sensitivity set inappropriately too high (e.g. -0.5 cmH$_2$O)
○ ↑ hemodynamic side effects because all breaths are delivered under (+ve) pressure

21.4.2 Synchronized intermittent mandatory ventilation (SIMV)

Description

- The patient receives preset No. of mandatory breaths (RR) of a preset V_T. Ventilator delivers mandatory breaths in synchrony with patient's inspiratory effort. If the ventilator does not detect an inspiratory effort within a certain time frame, the patient will receive a mandatory breath
- The patient can breathe spontaneously (at own generated volume) in between the mandatory breaths. Spontaneous breaths are often assisted with pressure support (PS)

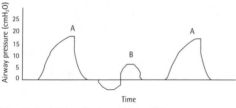

Fig. 41 Synchronized intermittent mandatory ventilation

Breath A: mandatory breaths
Breath B: spontaneous breath

Indications

- Normal respiratory drive, but unable to perform all of WOB
- Weaning (usually with PS)

Advantages

- Less atrophy of respiratory muscles than with AC mode
- Less hyperventilation/respiratory alkalosis than with AC mode
- Reduces hemodynamic adverse effects associated with AC because a part of V_E occurs at lower mean airway pressure (MAWP) due to the spontaneous breaths

Disadvantages

- May ↑ WOB at a low SIMV rate
- ↑ WOB for spontaneous breaths unless PS is added
- If the clinician sets RR too high, the patient may rely on set mandatory breaths and not breathe above the SIMV rate. This means that SIMV essentially becomes AC mode

Pressure-targeted:
(aka pressurecontrolled [PC] or pressure ventilation [PV])
Advantage: PIP constant with C_L, R_{aw} D = ↓ barotrauma risk
Caution: breath is P constant and V variable [↓ C_L or ↑ R_{aw} ⇒ ↓ V_T]

21.4.3 Pressure support (PS)

Description

- Preset inspiratory pressure augments each patient-triggered breath
- Inspiration ends when the flow ↓ to a certain level such as 25%
- Set to provide V_T of 5 - 8 ml/kg and RR < 25 bpm (full support = ≥ 20 cmH$_2$O)

Indications

- To overcome R_{aw} secondary to ETT + circuit in spontaneous breath (~ 5 - 8 cmH$_2$O)
- Weaning (possibly best weaning technique)
- May be used as initial mode of ventilation for moderate RF and adequate respiratory drive

Advantages

- Improves patient-ventilator synchrony (more physiological)
- ↓ WOB and ↓ respiratory muscle wasting
- ↓ barotrauma risk

Disadvantages

- Variable V_T [↓ C_L or ↑ Raw = ↓ V_T]
- May fail to trigger secondary to leak (cuff leak) because FR that ends PS breath is not reached
- Extra flow to circuit from external nebulizer may ⇒ asynchrony and hypoventilation because ventilator may be unable to detect inspiratory effort (MDI or AC mode during neb therapy avoids this problem)

21.4.4 Pressure control (PC)

Description

Patient receives preset RR at preset pressure (V_T variable)

Indications

- Rarely used
- May be used in ARDS patients requiring: PIP (> 50 cmH_2O), P_{plat} > 35 cmH_2O, PEEP > 15 cmH_2O; High FIO_2 during volume modes

Advantages

- ↓ Risk of barotrauma secondary to constant PIP
- Improves oxygenation as a result of ↑ MAWP

Disadvantages

- Variable V_T (need frequent pressure changes)
- Sedation/paralysis required

Dual control:
- Switch from V to P ventilation or vice versa within a breath or on a breath-to-breath basis
- May provide advantages of both V and P modes while avoiding their disadvantages

21.4.5 Pressure–regulated volume control (PRVC)

Description

Uses V_T as a feedback to continuously adjust minimum pressure needed to maintain set V_T (↓ C_L = ↑ pressure to deliver set V_T and vice versa)

Advantages

Can be used for initial ventilatory support (similar to AC, but with pressure monitoring)

Disadvantages

↓ Barotrauma risk as minimum PIP is used by the ventilator to achieve set V_T (ventilator calculates compliance)

21.4.6 Volume support (VS)

Description
Similar to PRVC and PS. Set V_T is used as feedback to adjust PS level
(VS = PS + guaranteed volume)

Advantages
Weaning

Disadvantages
$\downarrow C_L$ or $\uparrow R_{aw}$ = $\uparrow$ PS to maintain desired V_T and vice versa

21.5 Correcting Ventilation and Oxygenation in Response to Blood Gases

21.5.1 Hypoventilation ($\uparrow$ $PaCO_2$, $\downarrow$ pH)

$\downarrow V_E$ ($\downarrow V_T \pm \downarrow$ RR) = $\downarrow V_A$
- In volume ventilation:
  (a) $\uparrow V_T$ up to 10 - 12 ml/kg
  (b) $\uparrow$ RR (if V_T high and P_{plat} > 30 cmH$_2$0)
- In pressure ventilation:
  (a) $\uparrow$ set pressure (PIP)
  (b) $\uparrow$ Ti if short

$\uparrow$ **VCO_2: $\uparrow$ carbohydrates, trauma, sepsis, burns**
- Use high-fat, low-carbohydrate diet
- Correct underlying cause

$\uparrow$ **Deadspace: excess tubing, lung disease (PE, ARDS)**
- Remove V_D tubing: cut excess ETT at 2 cm from teeth
- Confirm diagnosis and treat

21.5.2 Hyperventilation ($\downarrow$ $PaCO_2$, $\uparrow$ pH)

1. VT $\pm$ RR set too high:
- In volume ventilation, $\downarrow$ RR, then $\downarrow V_T$ if necessary
- In pressure ventilation, $\downarrow$ RR, $\downarrow$ set pressure if necessary

2. ↑ Spontaneous RR: pain, anxiety, CNS problems, etc.:
- Sedation, anxiolytic agents, pain medications
- Add mechanical dead space ($V_D$mech) if head injury

3. Ventilator auto-cycling: adjust sensitivity

21.5.3 Under-oxygenation

1. $PaO_2 < 60$ mmHg, $SaO_2 < 90\%$: ↑ FIO_2, add or ↑ PEEP if $FIO_2 > 0.5$
2. ↑ V/Q mismatch or shunt: ARDS, pneumonia, atelectasis, pulmonary edema, etc.:
   Improve lung function: suction, bronchodilators, diuretics, antibiotics
3. Anemia and/or ↓ CO: optimize Hb (> 10 g/dl) ± CO

21.5.4 Over-oxygenation

- $PaO_2 > 100$ mmHg and SaO_2 100% on low FIO_2
- ↓ FIO_2 in 0.05 - 0.10 increments as tolerated, followed by ↓ PEEP

21.6 Monitoring Respiratory Mechanics

Monitoring changes in the trend (q shift or day) of airway pressures, compliance and airway pressures helps to evaluate the patient's condition and minimize ventilation-induced complications

21.6.1 Airway pressures

Peak Inspiratory Pressure
- PIP = highest pressure at end inspiration. It is the pressure that delivers V_T over resistance and lung stiffness
- PIP = P_{plat} + R_{aw}
- Persistent PIP > 45 - 50 cmH$_2$O = ↑ barotrauma risk
- ↑ PIP = ↓ C_L or ↑ R_{aw}
- ↓ PIP = improved C_L or R_{aw} or system leak

Plateau pressure (P_{plat})
- P_{plat} = pressure required to overcome C_L to deliver V_T. It reflects P_{alv}, so it is more important to follow than PIP
- Obtained by using inspiratory hold for ~ 1 second (no flow) ⇒ alveolar and mouth pressure equalize; therefore, P_{plat} ~ P_{alv}
- ↑ P_{plat} > 30 cmH$_2$O = ↑ barotrauma risk (may have to accept higher P_{plat} with ↓ chest wall compliance: scoliosis, abdominal distention)

21.6.2 Compliance

Static compliance (C_{st})
- Reflects lung/chest wall elasticity
- Equation: $C_{st} = V_T / (P_{plat} - PEEP)$
- Normal value: > 60 ml/cmH$_2$O
- Cst < 25 - 30 ml/cmH$_2$O = probable weaning failure
- ↓ **Cst** = lung parenchyma, pleural or chest wall disorders
- ↑ **Cst** = emphysema, improved lung parenchymal disease

Dynamic compliance (C_{dyn})
- Reflects Raw (measured during airflow) + lung/chest wall elasticity
- Equation: $C_{dyn} = V_T / (PIP - PEEP)$
- Normal value: 40 - 50 ml/cmH$_2$O (always < C_{st}, as PIP is always > P_{plat})
- ↓ **C_{dyn}** = ↓Cst or ↑R_{aw} (kinked tube, secretions, bronchospasm)
- ↑ **C_{dyn}** = ↑ Cst or ↓R_{aw}

21.6.3 Airway resistance (R_{aw})
- R_{aw} = airflow resistance caused by natural and artificial airway
- Airway resistance varies directly with length and inversely with airway diameter
  ↓ diameter by ½ = ↑R_{aw} by 16-fold (Poiseuille's Law)
- Normal value: 0.5 - 2.5 cmH$_2$O/L/s; (4 - 8 cmH$_2$O/L/s intubated)
- Equation: $R_{aw} = PIP - Pplat$
- ↑ **R_{aw}**: secretions, bronchospasm, small ETT, kinked tube, condensation or secretions in HME
- ↑ **R_{aw}**: ↑PIP, ↑PIP - P_{plat} difference and ↓ C_{dyn} with unchanged C_{st}

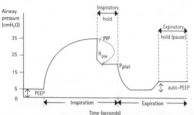

Fig. 42 Graphic representation of ventilator pressure - time waveform. It is showing various pressures that can be determined to help the clinician for better monitoring the patient's condition.

- **PEEP** = positive end-expiratory pressure (in this case it is 5 cmH$_2$O)
- **Auto-PEEP** = if we use expiratory hold at end exhalation we can determine if any auto-PEEP (air trapping) is present
- **PIP** = peak inspiratory pressure, which is the maximum pressure reached on inspiration
- **P$_{plat}$** = plateau pressure; approximates alveolar pressure; it is measured by using inspiratory hold at peak (end inspiration)
- **R$_{aw}$** = PIP – P$_{plat}$ = pressure needed to overcome airway resistance. This difference increases with increased R$_{aw}$

21.7 Ventilator Emergency and Troubleshooting

Sudden, severe distress:
High ± low pressure alarms sounding, dyspnea, cyanosis, (SpO$_2$ < 80 - 85%), diaphoresis, patient fighting ventilator

⇓

(1) Remove patient from ventilator and manually bag with 100% O$_2$

(2) Perform rapid assessment: vital signs, SpO$_2$, connections, appropriate settings

(3) Confirm airway placement and patency: look for adequate bilateral BS and chest rising, + if suction catheter passes easily

⇓	⇓
Distress remains = patient problem	**Distress improves = ventilator problem**
(1) ↑ Resistance to bagging (↑PIP, ↓ or absent BS ± inadequate chest rising) ⇓	(1) Leak/disconnection ⇓ Reconnect
• if cannot pass suction catheter, rule out bite/kinked tube	(2) Wrong settings: FIO$_2$, V$_E$, sensitivity, inadequate flow ⇓ **Set appropriately**
• if cannot ventilate (plugged and unable to suction), deflate cuff and **mask** ventilate = some air moves around ETT until reintubation possible	(3) Ventilator problem/inoperative ⇓ **Change ventilator**
• if ETT at carina or right main bronchus (↓BS and chest expansion on left): withdraw tube until bilateral BS	

(2) ↓ **Resistance to bagging**
(↓ PIP ± ↓ or no BS)
⇓
cuff leak ⇒ reinflate
extubated ⇒ reintubate

(3) Severe wheezing (↑ PIP)
⇓
bronchodilators, steroids, rule out
aspiration or CHF

21.7.1 Troubleshooting pressure alarms

↑ PIP, normal P_{plat} (= normal C_{st}, ↓ C_{dyn})
• ↑ secretions ⇒ suction
• Bronchospasm ⇒ give bronchodilator
• Kinked tube ⇒ unkink

↑ PIP, ↑ P_{plat} (= ↓ C_{st}, ↓ C_{dyn})
• PTX
• Atelectasis, ARDS
• Acute CHF/pulmonary edema
• ETT in right main bronchus

↓ PIP (= ↓ volume)
• Leak ⇒ correct
• Inadequate flow ⇒ ↑ flow
• Disconnection ⇒ reconnect
• Extubated ⇒ reintubate

21.8 Non-invasive Positive Pressure Ventilation (NPPV)

Background
1. Noninvasive positive pressure ventilation refers to the delivery of ventilatory support to the patient using techniques that do not require ETT
2. Interfaces used for the delivery of NPPV or CPAP

Nasal mask: used often, especially for chronic applications. Selecting the correct size is critical. The bottom of the mask should fit above the upper lip, while the top of the mask should lie slightly below the nasal bridge. If positioned too high, it will lead to air leak into the eyes. Choose smaller mask over larger so as to decrease air leak, in order to achieve good air seal. These masks often cause skin irritation and occasionally ulceration by exerting pressure over the bridge of the nose

Oronasal mask: covers both mouth and nose, leading to greater ventilation than with oronasal mask. These masks are mainly used on patients with acute respiratory failure (e.g. during first 24 hours of NPPV, then may change to nasal mask as the patient improves). Disadvantages: claustrophobic, decreased patient comfort and must be removed in order for the patient to eat, expectorate or speak

Nasal pillows: do not exert pressure over the bridge of the nose and may be preferred by the patients who suffer from claustrophobia

Total face mask: transparent mask that covers the whole face, resembling a hockey goalkeeper's mask

Indications

- Mild to moderate acute hypoxemic ± hypercapnic respiratory failure caused by acute exacerbations of COPD, CHF/pulmonary edema, obesity hypoventilation and possibly asthma
- Avoid intubation or reintubation in postoperative or post-extubation respiratory failure
- For patients who refuse intubation (e.g. end-stage lung disease)
- Chronic, long-term ventilation at home (BiPAP or CPAP) such as for obstructive sleep apnea (OSA) and neuromuscular disorders or chest wall deformities (e.g. kyphoscoliosis, ALS, muscular dystrophy, thoracoplasty)
- Weaning from invasive ventilation, when conventional weaning strategies fail

Contraindications

- Respiratory arrest
- Unable to protect upper airway and/or vomiting (risk of aspiration)
  - Impaired cough
  - Impaired swallowing
- Unable to follow commands (uncooperative) or tolerate facial mask
- Excessive secretions (unable to handle)
- Facial deformity, trauma, burns or surgery interfering with mask fit

- Medically unstable:
  - Hemodynamic instability (e.g. hypotensive shock)
  - Uncontrolled cardiac ischemia or arrhythmia
- Agitated or uncooperative
- Recent upper GI tract surgery
- Untreated PTX: intercostal drain should be inserted before commencing NPPV
- Life-threatening hypoxemia

Initial ventilator settings

NPPV can be delivered with ICU ventilator (preferred for hospital setting) because it provides consistent FIO_2 and allows for monitoring of V_T, RR, Ti and alarms OR portable bilevel pressure ventilators (preferred for long-term use) via nasal or face mask.

> NOTE: *Volumes vary because these are pressure-targeted modes.*

- **ICU ventilator:** pressure support (PS) or pressure control (PC):
  - **Inspiratory pressure:** 10 - 20 cmH_2O until $V_T \geq 7$ ml/kg & RR ≤ 25/min
  - **PEEP:** 0 - 6 cmH_2O
  - **Back-up RR:** 8 - 10 breaths/min

- **Bi-level pressure support** or **bi-level positive airway pressure (BiPAPâ):**
  - **Inspiratory positive airway pressure (IPAP):**
    8 - 12 cmH_2O; ↑ in increments of 2 cmH_2O until $V_T \geq 7$ ml/kg and RR ≤ 25/min; (IPAP = PS)
  - **Expiratory positive airway pressure (EPAP):**
    3 - 6 cmH_2O (EPAP = PEEP)
  - FIO_2: bleed in, titrate with SpO_2
  - Back-up RR: 10 breaths/min

- **Continuous positive airway pressure (CPAP):**
  - 5 - 12 cmH_2O
  - Applied from either CPAP valve connected to compressed gas source, small portable units such as those used for home therapy of obstructive sleep apnea (OSA) or critical care ventilators
  - CPAP may be of use for acute pulmonary edema because it decreases afterload, increases CO and of course increases oxygenation

NOTE: *Adjust setting as tolerated to alleviate dyspnea, decrease RR, increase V_T (if being monitored) and achieve good patient-ventilator synchrony. Provide oxygen to keep $SaO_2 > 90\%$. Monitor occasional ABGs within 1 - 2 hours of initiation on NPPV, 4 - 6 hours if the earlier sample showed little improvement and then as needed. Invasive ventilation should be considered if there is no improvement in $PaCO_2$ and pH, despite optimal ventilator settings. Pulse oximetry should be monitored for at least ≥ 24 hours after initiating NPPV.*

Advantages of NPPV over invasive ventilation
- Avoids complications of intubation/artificial airway
- Patient can eat, talk and be more in control
- ↓ Need for sedation

Adverse side effects and complications
- Mask related:
  - Skin breakdown, redness or ulceration of bridge of nose at points of contact with mask
  - Anxiety, claustrophobia
  - Discomfort, pain
- Air flow or pressure related:
  - Gastric distension (↑ risk if PIP > 20 - 25 cmH$_2$O)
  - Nasal dryness, sinus or ear pain, sleep arousal
- Air leak:
  - Need correct mask size
  - May compromise ventilation if patient is unable to compensate for the leak

BIBLIOGRAPHY

British Thoracic Society Guidelines: Non-invasive ventilation in acute respiratory failure, Thorax 2002; 57: 192-211.

Mehta S, Hill NS: Noninvasive ventilation, Am J Respir Crit Care Med 2001; 163: 540-577.

Hess DR, Kacmarek RM: Essentials of Mechanical Ventilation, 2nd ed. McGraw-Hill, 2002.

21.9 Weaning Mechanical Ventilation

Weaning = gradual discontinuation of MV

Quick withdrawal

Most patients (> 80%) need ventilatory support for < few days and can usually be simply disconnected (i.e. drug OD, anesthesia). There is no need for weaning

Gradual weaning

Required by patients with slowly resolving disease/process (e.g. severe trauma, bilateral pneumonia)

Unweanable

Some patients need long-term ventilatory support (i.e. ALS, muscular dystrophy)

21.9.1 Weaning check list

Initiate weaning when:
- Original problem (etiology of RF) is reversed or improved
- Stable CV system
- No infection (afebrile < 38°C)
- Adequate nutrition, sleep, electrolytes
- No sedation
- Optimal DO_2 (Hb $\geq$ 10 g/dl)
- Adequate oxygenation: $PaO_2 \geq 60$ mmHg on $FIO_2 \leq 0.4$

21.9.2 Weaning parameters

Purpose

To identify patients who are ready to breathe spontaneously and those who are not, in order to avoid premature weaning trials or prolonged mechanical ventilation and its associated complications.

Preferable

Easily measured parameters NOT requiring special equipment (i.e. RR, V_T, RR/V_T, V_E, ABG/pulse ox + signs of distress) + MIP and V_C for NM disease

21.9.3 Weaning predictors

Abbre-viations	Weaning index	Normal range	Weaning success?
Mechanics			
RR	Respiratory rate	10 - 20 breaths/min; up to $\geq$ 30 baseline in chronic restrictive lung disease	$\leq$ 25 - 30
MIP	Maximum inspiratory pressure	> 60 cmH$_2$O	> 25 - 30
V$_C$*	Vital capacity	60 - 75 ml/kg	> 10 - 15 (or >1L)
Cst	Static compliance	> 60 ml/cmH$_2$O	$\geq$ 30
P0.1*	Airway occlusion pressure in 0.1 second	< 2 cmH$_2$O	< 4 - 6
MVV*	Maximum voluntary ventilation	120 - 180 L/min	> 20 or $\geq$ 2 x V$_E$
Ventilation			
PaCO$_2$	Arterial carbon dioxide tension	35 - 45 mmHg up to 5 0 - 60 in COPD	< 50 $\leq$ 50 - 55 (COPD)
pH	Arterial blood pH	7.35 - 7.45	7.3 - 7.5
V$_T$	Tidal volume	5 - 8 ml/kg IBW	> 4 or $\geq$ 300 ml
V$_E$	Minute volume	5 - 8 L/min	< 10 - 12
V$_D$/V$_T$*	Dead space ventilation	25 - 40%	< 60%
Oxygenation			
PaO$_2$	Arterial O$_2$ tension	75 - 100 mmHg 55 - 65 (COPD)	> 60 - 70 on FIO$_2$ $\leq$ 0.40
SaO$_2$	Arterial O$_2$ saturation of Hb	> 95% (> 88 - 92 COPD)	> 90%
PaO$_2$/FIO$_2$	Arterial to inspired O$_2$ ratio	> 350	> 200

$P(A-a)O_2$	Alveolar to arterial O_2 tension gradient	5 - 25 mmHg on room air 25 - 65 on 100% O_2	< 350 on 100% O_2
PaO_2/P_AO_2	Arterial to alveolar O_2 tension ratio	0.85 - 0.95 (0.75 elderly)	> 0.35
Qs/Qt*	Shunt %	≤ 5%	< 20%
Hb	Hemoglobin	12 - 18 g/dl	> 8 - 10
Integrated indices			
RR/V_T	RR to V_T ratio; rapid shallow breathing index (RSBI)	40 - 60 breaths/min/L	< 100 - 105
CROP Index*	C = compliance (C_{dyn}) R = rate (RR) O = oxygenation (PaO_2/P_AO_2) P = pressure (MIP)	CROP = C_{dyn} x MIP x (PaO_2/P_AO_2)/RR	≥ 13 ml/breath/ min
SWI*	Simplified weaning index	SWI = RR (from vent) x (PIP - PEEP/MIP) x ($PaCO_2/40$)	< 9/min

*Not performed often, either because it requires patient cooperation and specialized equipment or it is too cumbersome.

21.9.4 ACCP/AARC/ACCM Evidence-Based Guidelines for Weaning and Discontinuing Ventilatory Support

A. Pathophysiology of ventilator dependence

Recommendation 1:

In patient requiring MV > 24 h, a search for all causes that may contribute to ventilator dependence should be undertaken. Reversing all possible ventilatory and nonventilatory issues should be an integral part of the ventilator discontinuation process.

B. Criteria to assess ventilator dependence

Recommendation 2:

Patients receiving MV for RF should be assessed for potential discontinuation if the following are satisfied:

1) Evidence for some reversal of the underlying cause of RF
2) Adequate oxygenation (and pH ≥ 7.25)
   a. $PaO_2/FIO_2 > 150 - 200$
   b. Requiring PEEP ≤ 5 - 8 cmH$_2$O and FIO$_2$ ≤ 0.4 - 0.5
3) Hemodynamic stability as defined by:
   a. Absence of active myocardial ischemia
   b. Absence of clinically important hypotension (i.e. no need for vasopressors or need for only low-dose vasopressors such as dopamine or dobutamine < 5 μg/kg/min)
4) Capable of initiating an inspiratory effort

The decision to use these criteria must be individualized. Some patients not satisfying all of the above criteria may be ready for attempts at discontinuation of MV.

Recommendation 3:

1) Discontinuation assessment should be performed during spontaneous breathing rather than while the patient is still receiving substantial ventilatory support. An initial brief period of spontaneous breathing can be used to assess the patient's ability to continue onto a formal spontaneous breathing trial (SBT)
2) The criteria with which to assess patient tolerance during SBT are:
   ○ Respiratory pattern: RR ≤ 30 - 35/min; spontaneous V_T ≥ 5 ml/kg
   ○ Adequate oxygenation: PaO_2 ≥ 60 mmHg on FIO$_2$ ≤ 0.4; PEEP ≤ 5-10 cmH$_2$O; PaO_2/FIO_2 ≥ 150 - 300; Hb ≥ 8 - 10 g/dl
   ○ Hemodynamic stability: HR ≤ 140/min; stable BP; no or minimal vasopressors
   ○ Subjective comfort
3) With tolerance of SBT lasting 30 - 120 min, consider permanent ventilator discontinuation

Criteria used to define tolerance in SBT

Objective measurements indicating tolerance/success:		
1	Acceptable gas exchange	$SpO_2 \geq 85 - 90\%$; $PaO_2 > 55 - 60$ mmHg; pH = 7.32; ↑ pH; $PaCO_2 \leq 10$ mmHg
2	Hemodynamic stability	HR < 120 - 140/min; HR not changed > 20%; sysBP < 180 - 200 mmHg and > 90 mmHg; BP not changed > 20% and no pressors required
3	Ventilatory pattern stable	RR ≤ 30 - 35/min; RR not changed > 50%
Subjective clinical assessment indicating intolerance/failure:		
1	Mental status changes	Somnolence, coma, agitation, anxiety
2	Signs of ↑ WOB	Accessory muscle use; thoracoabdominal paradox
3	Other	Diaphoresis; onset or worsening of discomfort

Recommendation 4:

Removal of artificial airway from a patient successfully weaned from MV should be based on assessment of airway patency and ability to protect the airway (good cough with airway suctioning)

1) Detection of air leak with ETT cuff deflated can be used to assess patency of upper airway (cuff leak test). A cuff leak < 110 ml during AC mode within 24 hours of extubation identifies a patient with ↑ risk for postextubation stridor

2) Postextubation stridor can be treated with steroids and/or epinephrine (± NIPPV, ± heliox) and do not necessarily need to be reintubated

Steroids ± epinephrine may be used 24 hours prior to extubation in patients with low cuff leak test

C. Managing the patient who has failed a spontaneous breathing trial

Recommendation 5:

Patients who fail an SBT should have the cause for failure determined. Once reversible causes for failed SBT are corrected and if the patient still meets the criteria in 3b (above), subsequent SBTs should be performed every 24 hours.

Recommendation 6:

Patients who fail an SBT should receive a stable, non-fatiguing, comfortable form of ventilatory support.

Recommendation 7:

Anesthesia/sedation strategies and ventilator management aimed at early extubation should be used in postsurgical patients.

Recommendation 8:

Weaning/discontinuing protocols designed for non-physician medical staff should be developed and implemented by ICUs. Protocols aimed at optimizing sedation should also be developed and implemented. There is clear evidence that non-physician (e.g. respiratory therapist-driven) protocols enhance clinical outcomes and reduce the costs.

> **NOTE**: Protocols should not be used to replace clinical judgement, but rather to complement it.

D. Role of tracheostomy in ventilator-dependent patients

Recommendation 9:

Tracheotomy should be considered after an initial period of stabilization on the ventilator, when it is apparent that the patient will require prolonged ventilator assistance. Patients who benefit from early tracheostomy include:

1) Those requiring high levels of sedation to tolerate translaryngeal tubes
2) Those with marginal respiratory mechanics (often manifested as tachypnea), in whom a tracheostomy tube having lower resistance might ↓ risk of muscle overload
3) Those who may derive psychological benefit from the ability to eat orally, communicate by articulated speech and experience enhanced mobility; and
4) Those in whom enhanced mobility may assist physical therapy efforts

E. The role of long-term facilities

Recommendation 10:

Unless there is evidence for clearly irreversible disease (e.g. high spinal cord injury or advanced ALS), a patient requiring MV for RF should not be considered permanently ventilator-dependent until 3 months of weaning attempts have failed.

Recommendation 11:

Critical care practitioners should familiarize themselves with facilities in their communities or in units in the hospitals they staff that specialize in managing patients who require prolonged dependence on MV. Such familiarization should include reviewing published peer-reviewed data from those units, if available. When medically stable for transfer, patients who have failed ventilator discontinuation attempts in the ICU should be transferred to those facilities that have demonstrated success and safety in accomplishing ventilator discontinuation.

Recommendation 12:
Weaning strategies in the prolonged mechanical ventilation patient should be slow paced and should include gradually lengthening self-breathing trials.

"Evidence-Based Guidelines for Weaning and Discontinuing Ventilatory Support" by:
ACCP: American College of Chest Physicians
AARC: American Association for Respiratory Care
ACCM: American College of Critical Care Medicine; published in:
Chest 2001; 12: 375-395S
Respir Care 2002; 47: 69-90

21.9.5 Weaning techniques

T-piece

The patient breathes humidified O_2 via T-piece connected to ETT for increasing periods. Between trials, the patient is connected back to ventilator and given full ventilatory support (AC mode). A T-piece can be created through the ventilator by using ~ 5 cmH_2O of PS, which eliminates R_{aw} from the ETT/ventilator circuit and provides alarms; there is thus no need for constant monitoring as is the case if the patient is disconnected from the ventilator.

SIMV + PS

Mandatory rate is gradually ↓ by 2 - 4 breaths/min as tolerated (RR < 25/min, ABG/pulse oximetry) and PS of ~ 5 - 8 cmH_2O is used to support spontaneous breaths and alleviate resistance caused by ETT/ventilatory circuit. Once SIMV rate of ~ 4 - 6 breaths/min is tolerated, consider extubation if indicated.

PS

Set PS so that V_T ~ 5 - 8 ml/kg and RR < 25/min. ↓ PS in increments of ~ 2 cmH_2O as long as tolerated. Once PS of 5 - 7 cmH_2O and patient tolerates it, consider extubation. PS may be the most effective weaning method (physiologic, comfortable), especially in slow weaning.

21.9.6 Signs and causes of weaning failure

Causes of failure

- ↓ **Muscle strength:** malnutrition, NM disease, sedatives, low Mg^{++}, K^+, $PO4^-$
- ↑ **WOB:**
  - ↑ R_{aw}: small ETT, obstruction, bronchospasm
  - ↓ C_L: atelectasis, obesity, ARDS
  - ↑ VCO_2: fever, high-carbohydrate diet

- **Hypoxemia:** lung disease, $\downarrow DO_2$ secondary to anemia, CHF

Signs of failure
- **Respiratory:** RR > 30 - 35/min, V_T < 4 ml/kg or < 275 ml, RR/V_T > 100 - 105 breaths/min/L, MIP < 20 cmH_2O, C_{st} < 25 ml/cmH_2O
- **ABG:** PaO_2 < 50 - 60 mmHg and SaO_2 < 85 - 90%, $\uparrow PaCO_2$ > 10 mmHg from baseline (> 50 - 55), pH < 7.3
- **Cardiovascular:** BP change by > 20%; HR change by 20%, arrhythmias
- **Other:** dyspnea, diaphoresis, cyanosis, accessory muscle use

---

21.9.7   Extubation

To extubate, patient must have:
- Good cough and gag reflex (stimulate with suction catheter)
- Large air leak with cuff deflated (indicates upper airway patency)
- No excess secretions, if patient cannot protect upper airway (inadequate cough/ gag reflex, excessive secretions), patient probably needs tracheostomy tube

Procedure
- Explain procedure to patient and have him/her sit in semi-Fowler position
- Preoxygenate, deflate cuff, suction ETT and loosen tape supporting ETT
- Withdraw ETT: ask patient to cough, to help force secretions into mouth
- Give similar FIO_2 as on ventilator via aerosol mask and encourage coughing and incentive spirometry (IS)

Complications and possible solutions

Postextubation stridor:
May be due to glottic edema or tracheal stenosis. Nebulized racemic epinephrine ± steroids should be administered to $\downarrow$ inflammation

Swallowing dysfunction:
May be due to ETT or NG tube. To protect against aspiration, have patient on nothing by mouth (NPO) for ≥ 24 hours

Excessive secretions: suction, CPT, bronchodilators

BIBLIOGRAPHY

Raoof S: Weaning From Mechanical Ventilation. In, Raoof S, Khan FA (eds): Mechanical Ventilation Manual, American College of Physicians, 1998.

Epstein SK: Weaning From Mechanical Ventilation, Respir Care 2002; 47: 454-466.

Pilbeam S: Mechanical Ventilation: Physiological and Clinical Applications, 3rd ed. Mosby, 1998.

Manthous CA, Schmidt GA, Hall JB: Liberation From Mechanical Ventilation, Chest 1998; 114: 886-901.

21.10 Adjuncts/Non-Conventional Techniques

21.10.1 Inverse ratio ventilation (IRV)

Description: strategy where Ti > Te (~ 2 : 1)

Indications

- Rarely used since there is no definitive proof that it is better than conventional ventilation with PEEP
- ARDS patients requiring > 50 cmH$_2$O and refractory hypoxemia to high FIO$_2$ and high PEEP may benefit from it

Techniques

Provided with pressure control (PC-IRV) or volume control (V$_C$-IRV)

Complications

Very uncomfortable = need sedation/paralysis

21.10.2 Permissive hyperkapnea

Description

'Lung protective strategy' intended to ↓ the incidence of alveolar overdistension and ventilator-induced lung injury, which may help avoid barotrauma or volutrauma caused by: excessive PIP, P$_{plat}$ and high V$_T$

Possible Indications
- When unable to achieve normal oxygenation and ventilation with $FIO_2 < 0.60$, PIP < 30 - 35 cmH_2O above PEEP
- May be considered for **ARDS** and **severe asthma** patients

Strategy

Low V_T (≤ 5 ml/kg) is used to keep $P_{plat} < 30$ cmH_2O and ↓ PIP while $PaCO_2$ is allowed to ↑ gradually to 60 - 100 mmHg (~ 10 mmHg/h) as long as the pH is ≥ 7.20

21.10.3 Positional therapy

Prone position
- May improve oxygenation in ARDS patients due to better V/Q matching when compared to supine position. Heart, large vessels and abdominal contents become dependent and do not push, on lungs as is the case with supine position
- **Risks:** accidental extubation, hemodynamic instability, removal of catheters or line and body injury
- **Contraindications:** spinal cord problems, cardiac problems, thoracic or abdominal surgery

Lateral position
- Placing 'good lung' down may improve oxygenation in unilateral lung disease
- Contraindications: lung abscess, pulmonary hemorrhage

21.10.4 Independent lung ventilation (ILV)

Description
- Gas is delivered to each lung by 2 ventilators via double lumen ETT
- Different parameters can be used for each lung
- **Double lumen ETT:**
  - Usually left angled double-lumen ETT is used because right angled double-lumen ETT is more difficult to place without obstructing right upper lobe (RUL)
  - Proximal cuff is located in trachea and distal cuff is located in bronchus

Indications
- Unilateral lung disease
- Massive hemoptysis
- Bronchopleural fistula
- Single lung transplant

Complications
- Tube migration
- Lumen is < ½ diameter of regular ETT which ⇒
  ○ Difficulty in spontaneous breathing, suctioning or bronchoscopy
  ○ Should change to regular ETT before weaning

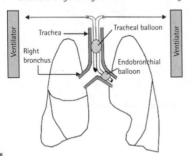

Fig. 43 Shows the correct placement of a left angled double-lumen tube

21.10.5 Liquid ventilation

Description
- 'Partial liquid ventilation - PLV' is the most common experimental technique
- Uses **perfluorocarbon** (PFC), a colorless, odorless, inert liquid as O_2-carrying fluid
- PFC has strong affinity for gases, lower surface tension than water

Administration
- Instilled into lungs via side port ETT without interrupting mechanical ventilation
- Instilled until meniscus seen in ETT ≈ FRC
- Add as needed to replace quickly evaporating liquid

Possible indications
ARDS/IRDS, pneumonia

Advantages

Acts as 'liquid PEEP' $\Rightarrow$
- Improved oxygenation
- Enhances clearance of secretions/debris that float on top of mucus because PFC is 2x heavier than water
- Reduces lung injury and enhances lung healing following debris removal

Complications
- Possible mucus plugs due to mobilized mucus and alveolar debris
- PFC is radiopaque, so similar densities may not be seen on CXR

BIBLIOGRAPHY

Kacmarek RK: Ventilatory Adjuncts, Respir Care 2002; 47; 319-330.

Hess DR, Kacmarek RM: Essentials of Mechanical Ventilation, 2nd ed. McGraw-Hill, 2002.

Multz AS: Liquid Ventilation. Respir Care Clin 2000; 6: 645-658.

Foley DS, Hirschl RB: Liquid Ventilation. In, MacIntyre NR, Branson RD (eds). Mechanical Ventilation. WB Saunders, 2001.

Pilbeam S: Mechanical Ventilation: Physiological and Clinical Applications, 3rd ed. Mosby , 1998.

21.11 Neonatal-Pediatric Ventilatory Support

21.11.1 Indications

Neonates
- Respiratory failure: $PaCO_2 > 55$ mmHg, pH < 7.20, $PaO_2 < 50$ mmHg on $FIO_2 > 0.60$ $\pm$ CPAP > 10 cmH_2O
- Apnea (unresponsive to CPAP), RDS, MAS, pneumonia, PPHN, CDH, sepsis, shock, CNS depression (drugs, trauma, intracranial hemorrhage [ICH]), congenital heart defects, premature infants with respiratory distress

Pediatrics
- Respiratory failure: $PaCO_2 > 50$ mmHg, pH < 7.25 - 7.30, $PaO_2 > 70$ mmHg on O_2
- NM disease, pneumonia, asthma, head trauma ($\uparrow$ICP)

NOTE: *Signs and symptoms of RF: persistent RR > 80/min in neonates and > 50/min in child, cyanosis, nasal flaring, grunting, retractions, poor air entry.*

21.11.2 Ventilator settings

NOTE: *Children weighing < 10 kg are often ventilated with pressure-limited ventilators (PIP is set instead of V_T); > 10 kg ventilated with volume-cycled ventilator (V_T is set).*

Tidal volume
Delivered ~ 5 - 8 ml/kg; adequate V_T = good chest excursion and good BS; children < 8 years of age, ventilated with uncuffed ETT (small leak up to 15% is acceptable)

Peak inspiratory pressure
Initial: good chest expansion + BS while BMV ≈ 15 - 20 cmH$_2$O to deliver V_T of ~ 5 - 8 ml/kg in neonates and 7 - 10 ml/kg in children; ↓ **compliance (RDS):** > 25 - 30 cmH$_2$O; as compliance improves, ↓PIP to avoid high V_T and risk of volu-/barotrauma

Respiratory rate
Term: 20 - 30/min; LBW: 30 - 40/min; > 10 kg weight: 8 - 14/min

Flow rate
5 - 12 L/min for neonates, higher in children; minimum FR = 2 x V_E

Inspiratory time
Neonate: 0.3 - 0.5 s (RDS 0.25 s); set so that I : E ratio is ~ 1 : 2

FIO$_2$
Minimum to keep baby **pink** and SpO$_2$ > 92%;
Lowest FIO$_2$ to keep PaO$_2$ 50 - 70 mmHg in premature baby, 60 - 80 mmHg in infant and 80 - 100 mmHg for child; if patient already on O$_2$ ± CPAP, may start at same level

PEEP
Start at 3 cmH$_2$O and ↑ in 2 cmH$_2$O increments to achieve PaO$_2$ 50 - 80 mmHg; ideal lung volume expansion = 8 - 9 ribs bilaterally on CXR (if diaphragm flat below rib 9 = PEEP is excessive); > 8 - 10 cmH$_2$O rarely used in neonates

Mean airway pressure

NOT set; = average pressure over entire respiratory cycle; maintain < 12 cmH$_2$O to ↓ barotrauma risk; ↑ MAWP = ↑ oxygenation; increases from: ↑ PIP, PEEP, V$_T$, RR, FR and Ti

Mode

- **Synchronized intermittent mandatory ventilation:** preferred over AC for neonates/small children
- **Assist control:** not used often in neonates/small children because of poor response time with high RR ⇒ asynchrony, ↑ effort to trigger breath
- **Pressure support:** may be used alone in reliable respiratory drive or with SIMV

21.11.3 Adjusting ventilation and oxygenation

Adjusting ventilation	
To ↑ ventilation (↓ PaCO$_2$)	**To ↓ ventilation (↑ PaCO$_2$)**
• ↑ Respiratory rate • ↑ PIP up to 25 - 30 cmH$_2$O (or ↑ V$_T$)	• ↓ Peak inspiratory pressure (PIP) • ↓ Respiratory rate
Adjusting oxygenation	
To ↑ oxygenation (↑ PaO$_2$)	**To ↓ oxygenation (↓ PaO$_2$)**
• ↑ FIO$_2$ up to 0.5 - 0.6 • ↑ PEEP up to 10 cmH$_2$O • ↑ RR and Ti (↑ V$_T$ in vol-modes)	• ↓ FIO$_2$ • ↓ PEEP • ↓ MAWP

21.11.4 Weaning

Indications

- Condition requiring mechanical ventilation is reversed/stabilized
- Acceptable ABG + FIO$_2$ < 0.5 and PEEP < 8 cmH$_2$O

Methods

- **SIMV:**
  - ↓ **PIP** in increments of 2 cmH$_2$O
  - ↓ **RR** in increments of 2/min
  - ↓ **FIO$_2$** to 0.40 in 2% increments
  - ↓ **PEEP** to 5 cmH$_2$O in increments of 1 cmH$_2$O

- **PS:** ↓ in ~ 2 cmH$_2$O increments as long as V$_T$ stays ~ 5 - 7 ml/kg and no significant ↑ RR with each ↓ PS level
- **CPAP:** common among pediatric patients; may use CPAP trial prior to extubation; may initiate when: PIP < 25 cmH$_2$O, RR < 15/min, FIO$_2$ < 0.40, PEEP < 5 cmH$_2$O; LBW infants may not tolerate CPAP via ETT because of the ↑ WOB through small ETT - may do better if extubated and given O$_2$ by oxyhood [↑ FIO$_2$ by 10 - 20% > on ventilator]

21.11.5 Extubation

- Consider when:
  - PIP ≤ 15 - 18 cmH$_2$O
  - PEEP ≤ 5 cmH$_2$O
  - RR ≤ 12/min and
  - FIO$_2$ ≤ 0.30 - 0.40
- Audible leak should be present. If no leak, assume laryngeal edema is present and treat with racemic epinephrine ± steroids before extubation
- **Postextubation:**
  - Maintain oxygenation with oxyhood, nasal CPAP or nasal cannula?
  - With signs of edema/subglottic stenosis, give racemic epinephrine ± dexamethasone

21.11.6 High frequency ventilation

Description

HFV uses RR > 150/min and V$_T$ ≤ V$_D$. It is mostly used with neonates. There are several techniques available, of which **high frequency jet ventilation (HFJV)** and **high frequency oscillation (HFO)** are the most common. Major advantage of HFV: adequate oxygenation/ventilation at lower PIP and MAWP than conventional ventilation

Indications

- Rescue therapy for patients failing conventional ventilation ± complications (high PIP)
- Diseases treated:
  - IRDS
  - CDH
  - PPHN
  - MAS

- Bronchopleural fistula
- PTX
- Upper airway or lung surgery

Possible complications
- Air trapping
- Tracheitis due to high jet flow ± inadequate humidity
- Hypotension
- Decreased CO and
- Pulmonary overdistension

21.11.7 Techniques

High frequency oscillation

Description:
Alternate positive and negative pressure ⇒ gas is pushed in and pulled out of the lungs. This means that inspiration and expiration is active

Initial settings:
- **RR or frequency (f):** 180 - 1200/min (3 - 15 Hz)
  - Neonate < 2 kg: 12 - 15 Hz
  - Neonate > 2 kg: 8 - 10 Hz
- **V_T:** ≤ 1 - 3 ml/kg (< V_D)
- **Inspiratory time percent (Ti%):** 0.33 sec (I:E ratio ~ 1:1). Expiration is active
- **PEEP:** same as conventional ventilator
- **FIO_2:** 0.21 - 1.0
- **MAWP:** ~ 2 cmH_2O > MAWP on conventional ventilator
- **Drive pressure (DP) or amplitude:** ~ 2 cmH_2O < PIP on conventional ventilator: adequate to achieve chest wall vibration (wiggle)
- **Bias flow:** 10 - 20 L/min

High frequency jet ventilation

Description:
HFJV is used with conventional ventilator. HFJV delivers high pressure jets of gas via small catheter placed inside ETT, special triple-lumen ETT or special jet adaptor placed on ETT.

Initial settings:
- **RR or f:** 150 - 660/min (2.5 - 11 Hz)
  - Premature: 440 - 660/min
  - Full term: 300 - 420/min
  - Children: 240 - 320/min
- **V_T:** 2 - 5 ml/kg ($\leq V_D$)
- **Ti%:** 0.33 sec (I:E ~ 1:1 - 1:2)
- **PEEP:** same as conventional ventilator
- **FIO$_2$:** 0.21 - 1.0

Things to consider:
- **Adequate inflation** = lung volume on CXR at ribs T8 - T9 + chest wall wiggle
- **Suctioning:** if possible should be avoided in 1st 24 hours of HFV. Indicated when there is ↓ chest wall movement or there are visible/audible secretions in the airway

Weaning:
- ↓ FIO$_2$ to < 0.40
- ↓ MAWP in 1 - 2 cmH$_2$O increments
- ↓ change of pressure (DP) in ~ 4 cmH$_2$O increments
- May switch to conventional ventilator when MAWP < 10 cmH$_2$O and FIO$_2$ is < 0.50 + acceptable ABG

BIBLIOGRAPHY

Meredith KS: High-Frequency Ventilation. In, Czervinske MP, Barnhart (eds): Perinatal and Pediatric Respiratory Care. WB Saunders, 2003.

MacIntyre NR: High-Frequency Ventilaton. In, MacIntyre NR, Branson RD (eds): Mechanical Ventilation. WB Saunders, 2001.

21.11.8 Extracorporal membrane oxgenation

Description
- ECMO is a temporary 'last-resort' heart-lung bypass for neonates
  ± children with severe respiratory failure that is nonresponsive to conventional ventilation and therapy
- It is used to 'rest' the lungs and provide oxygenation outside of the body while the lung is healing
- ECMO circuit:
  - **Cannulas** for blood drainage and reinfusion
  - Blood **pump**
  - Membrane **oxygenator** for O_2 and CO_2 exchange
  - **Heat exchanger** for rewarming blood before reinfusion
  - Tubing and various connectors

Types of ECMO circuits
Venoarterial (VA) ECMO:
- Venous blood is drained from right atrium (RA) via internal jugular vein; it passes through oxygenator (where O_2 is added and CO_2 is removed) and returns to arterial circulation via right common artery
- V_A ECMO provides support for **both** heart and lungs

Venovenous (VV) ECMO:
- Venous blood is drawn from RA via catheter placed in internal jugular vein; it passes through ECMO circuit, where it is oxygenated and returns to RA via inferior vena cava
- VV ECMO **only** provides lung support; therefore, it is reserved for patients with adequate CO

Indications
- Severe **reversible** cardiac ± respiratory failure when maximum therapy is ineffective
- Diseases treated: MAS, CDH, sepsis, PPHN, IRDS, pneumonia, heart failure

- Criteria:
  - ◦ > 34-week gestation age ± > 2 kg weight
  - ◦ Mechanical ventilation used for < 7 - 10 days
  - ◦ No ICH, congenital or major cardiac disease
  - ◦ Oxygenation index (OI) > 40 for 4 hours
    $$OI = (MAWP \times FIO_2) / (PaO_2 \times 100)$$
  - ◦ No serious bleeding/untreatable coagulopathy

Complications
- ↑ Risk for infections (invasive)
- Technical failure: pump, cannula, tubing, oxygenator
- Seizures, pulmonary hemorrhage, intraventricular hemorrhage
- Bleeding due to overuse of heparin
- Clots due to underuse of heparin

BIBLIOGRAPHY

Gentile MA, Cheifetz IM: Extracorporeal Techniques for Cardiopulmonary Support. In, MacIntyre NR, Branson RD (eds.): Mechanical Ventilation. WB Saunders, 2001.

Hansell DR: Extracorporeal Membrane Oxygenation for Perinatal and Pediatric Patients, Respir Care 2003; 48: 352-362Hess DR, Kacmarek RM: Essentials of Mechanical Ventilation, 2nd ed. McGraw-Hill, 2002.

Pilbeam S: Mechanical Ventilation: Physiology and Clinical Applications, 3rd ed. Mosby, 1998.

Raoof S, Khan F: Mechanical Ventilation Manual, American College of Physicians, 1998.

22. Pulmonary Procedures

22.1 Arterial Puncture/Cannulation

Radial artery is preferred site for arterial blood sampling because
- It is near the surface and is easy to palpate
- Collateral circulation normally exists in ulnar artery
- It is not near any large veins
- It is relatively pain free
- Brachial artery is the next choice when unable to palpate radial artery (e.g. weak pulse) or with -ve Allen test. **Femoral artery** is usually reserved for emergency (e.g. during CPR)

Steps
1. Perform a modified Allen test to assess for adequate collateral circulation
   a. Ask the patient to make a fist, then apply pressure with fingers to both radial and ulnar arteries. Blanching of the palm and fingers should occur
   b. Ask the patient to open the hand and remove pressure on ulnar artery. This should result in flushing of entire hand in < 10 seconds
   c. If there is no flushing of the hand, the Allen test is -ve (ulnar artery is not patent) and the other hand should be tried before attempting brachial artery puncture

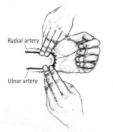

Radial artery

Ulnar artery

Fig. 44 Modified Allen Test

2. Clean the site with 70% isopropyl alcohol, heparinize the syringe and expel the excess

3. Palpate and secure the artery with one hand and slowly insert the needle bevel up (20 – 22 gauge for adults, 23 – 25 gauge for children/infants) at 30 – 45° angle until blood pulsates into the syringe

4. Allow 2 – 4 ml of blood to fill the syringe, pull out the needle and apply firm pressure with other hand to the puncture site with sterile gauze until bleeding stops (~ 3 – 5 min, longer if necessary). The patient may be able to do this step while you perform the rest of the procedure

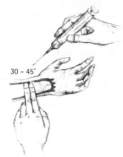

30 – 45°

Fig. 45 Arterial puncture technique

5. Expel any air bubbles and cap/plug the syringe and place it in ice (if unable to process sample within 15 – 20 min). Chilled samples should be discarded if not analyzed within 60 min

6. Dispose of waste materials/sharps appropriately and document the procedure and patient status.

> **NOTE 1:** *Rarely, a local anesthetic (1 – 2% lidocaine) may need to be injected sub-cutaneously and periarterially before arterial puncture (wait 2 min for effect) to ↓ anxiety-related changes in blood gas values and/or for arterial cannulation.*
>
> **NOTE 2:** *Never recap used needle without a safety device, never handle it using both hands and never point it toward any part of the body/other people present.*

Complications

Nerve damage, thrombus formation, infection and bleeding/hematoma

22.2 Radial Arterial Cannulation

Indications

1. Need for precise and continuous measurement of arterial blood pressure (e.g. hypertensive crisis, shock)

2. Need for frequent ABG analysis

Contraindications

Relative contraindications include bleeding diathesis, anticoagulants or thrombolytic use.

Insertion technique

1. The procedure is the same as when performing arterial puncture, except that the catheter is inserted directly into the artery over a needle

2. The needle is pulled out gently while the catheter is slightly advanced into the artery

3. Attach the arterial monitoring apparatus (transducer, tubing and pressure bag with preheparinized saline) and secure the catheter into place with transparent tape

NOTE: *Some clinicians use arm board with a gauze roll behind the wrist to hyperextend the joint for more stability.*

BIBLIOGRAPHY

Scanlan CL, Wilkins RL: Analysis and Monitoring of Gas Exchange. In, Wilkins RL, Stoller JK, Scanlan CL (eds): Egan's Fundamentals of Respiratory Care, 8th ed. Mosby, 2003.

Singer M, Webb A: Oxford Handbook of Critical Care. Oxford University Press, 1997.

22.3   Pulmonary Artery Catheter

Indications

- Diagnosis of shock states, PPH, valvular disease, PE, intracardiac shunts (e.g. ASD, VSD) and right heart failure
- ARDS
- To measure PAWP, vascular resistance (SVR, PVR), SvO_2, CO and calculate variables such as VO_2, DO_2, O_2ER and shunt fraction
- Assess response to therapies
- When PEEP > 10 - 15 cmH_2O is needed during invasive positive pressure ventilation (IPPV)
- Temporary pacing
- To differentiate low versus high pressure pulmonary edema

Insertion technique

Inserted into a major vein (jugular, subclavian or femoral). Right internal jugular vein approach is described below; it is the shortest path to the heart.

- **Preinsertion:** check the catheter as per manufacturer's recommendations (e.g. check for cracks, balloon function), place transparent sleeve over the catheter to maintain sterility, connect all lumens to stopcocks and flush them to eliminate air bubbles
- Internal jugular vein is cannulated with a needle through which a flexible wire is introduced into the vein. Remove the needle and place introducer over the wire, then withdraw the wire and pass the PA catheter through the introducer
- With the PA catheter ~ 15 cm into the vein, inflate the balloon with 1 - 1.5 ml and allow catheter tip to be floated by the bloodstream through the right heart and into pulmonary artery, while observing for changes in waveform on the monitor
- Once a characteristic PAWP waveform is obtained, note the pressure and deflate the balloon (to avoid pulmonary infarct); this leads to return of PA waveform. From the right internal jugular vein approach:
  - **RA waveform** is observed when ~ 25 - 30 cm of PA catheter has been advanced into the vein
  - **RV waveform** occurs at ~ 30 - 40 cm
  - **PA waveform** occurs at ~ 40 - 45 cm
  - **PAWP occurs** at ~ 45 - 55 cm
  - Obtain CXR to confirm catheter's position and exclude PTX

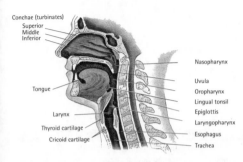

Fig. 46 Characteristics of quadruple pulmonary artery (Swan-Ganz) catheter. Distal port is used for measurement of pulmonary artery pressure and aspiration of mixed venous blood; proximal port is located about 30 cm from the tip and is used for central venous pressure (right arterial pressure) monitoring and fluid infusion; thermistor lumen is ~ 4 cm proximal to the balloon and is used for measuring temperature changes for cardiac output calculation (thermodilution)

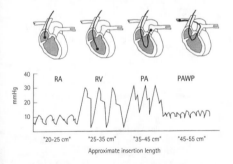

Fig. 47 Position of the pulmonary artery catheter as it is advanced through the heart and wedged in the pulmonary artery

Complications
- PTX
- Hemorrhage
- Cardiac arrhythmias
- Infection (bacteremia, endocarditis)
- Thrombosis
- Rupture of pulmonary artery
- Cardiac perforation
- Injury to cardiac valves (do not withdraw catheter unless balloon is deflated)
- Pulmonary infarction

Hemodynamic parameters

Parameter		Formula	Normal value
Measured variables			
MABP	Mean arterial blood pressure	MABP = sysBP + (2 x diaBP)/3	70 - 100 mmHg
PAP	Pulmonary artery pressure	MPAP = sysPAP + (2 x diaPAP)/3	MPAP: 15 - 18 mmHg diaPAP: 5 - 12 mmHg sysPAP: 15 - 25 mmHg
PAWP	Pulmonary artery wedge pressure	A measure of LA (> 18 = impending pulmonary edema; > 30 = acute pulmonary edema)	4 - 12 mmHg
RAP	Right atrial pressure	Central venous pressure (CVP)	0 - 8 mmHg
RVP	Right ventricular pressure	RVSP: right ventricular systolic pressure RVDP: right ventricular diastolic pressure	15 - 30 mmHg 0 - 5 mmHg
CO	Cardiac output	CO = HR x SVCO = $VO_2/(CaO_2 - CvO_2)$ x 10	4 - 8 L/min 0.6 - 0.8 L/min (newborn)

Calculated variables			
CI	Cardiac index	$CI = CO/BSA$	$2.5 - 4 \ L/min/m^2$
SV	Stroke volume	$SV = CO/HR$	$60 - 120 \ ml$
SI	Stroke index	$SI = SV/HR$	$40 - 60 \ ml/beat/m^2$
SVR	Systemic vascular resistance	$SVR = (MABP - CVP)/CO \times 80$	$900 - 1500 \ dynes/sec/cm^{-5}$
PVR	Pulmonary vascular resistance	$PVR = (MPAP - PAWP)/CO \times 80$	$25 - 200 \ dynes/sec/cm^{-5}$
LVSWI	Left ventricular stroke work index	$LVSWI = SI \times (MABP - PAWP) \times 0.0136$	$45 - 60 \ g/beat/m^2$
RVSWI	Right ventricular stroke work index	$RVSWI = SI \times (MPAP - CVP) \times 0.0136$	$5 - 10 \ g/beat/m^2$
DO_2	Oxygen delivery	$DO_2 = CI \times 10 \times CaO_2$	$500 - 750 \ ml/min/m^2$
VO_2	Oxygen consumption	$VO_2 = (CaO_2 - CvO_2) \times CI \times 10$	$100 - 180 \ ml/min/m^2$
CaO_2	Arterial blood oxygen content	$CaO_2 = (1.34 \times Hb \times SaO_2) + (PaO_2 \times 0.003)$	$16 - 20 \ ml/dl$
CvO_2	Mixed venous oxygen content	$CvO_2 = (1.34 \times Hb \times SvO_2) + (PvO_2 \times 0.003)$	$12 - 15 \ ml/dl$
$C(a-v)O_2$	Difference between CaO_2 and CvO_2	$CaO_2 - CvO_2$	$3 - 5.5 \ ml/dl$
O_2ER	Oxygen extraction ratio	$O_2ER = VO_2/DO_2$	$20 - 30\%$

NOTE: *Values may vary significantly depending on person's fitness and disease.*

Hemodynamic changes In various disorders

Pathology	CVP	PAP	PAWP	COP	VR	SVR
ARDS	N/↑	N/↑	N	N	↑	N
COPD	N/↑	↑	N	N/↓	↑	N/↓
Heart failure						
LVF	N/↑	↑	↑	↓	↑	↑
RVF (cor pulmonale)	↑	N	N/↓	↓	N	N/↑
Hypovolemia	↓	↓	↓	↓	N	↑
Hypervolemia	↑	↑	↑	↑	N	N/↓
MI	N/↑	N/↑	N/↑	↓	N/↑	↑↓
Pulmonary edema/CHF	N	↑	↑	N/↓	↑	↑↓
Pulmonary embolism	↑	↑	N/↓	N/↓	↑	N
Shock						
Cardiogenic	N/↑	↑	↑	↓	N/↑	↑
Septic	N	N/↑	N/↑	↓	N/↑	↑↓
Valvular						
Mitral valve stenosis	N	↑	↑	N/↓	N/↑	N/↑
Aortic valve stenosis	N/↑	↑	↑	↓	↑	↑

NOTE: *Significant variations may exist. [Key: N = normal; / = or].*

BIBLIOGRAPHY

Philip JF: The Pulmonary Artery Catheter. In, Parsons PE, Heffner JE (eds): Pulmonary/Respiratory Therapy Secrets, 2nd ed. Hanley & Belfus, 2002.

Singer M, Webb A: Oxford Handbook of Critical Care. Oxford University Press, 1997.

Chan ED et al: Bedside Critical Care Manual, 2nd ed. Hanley & Belfus, 2002.

22.4 Thoracocentesis

Indications
- Diagnostic 'tap' to determine the etiology of a pleural effusion (> 10 mm of free-flowing fluid on lateral decubitus CXR)
- Analysis of pleural fluid in the diagnosis staging of suspected/known malignancy
- Symptomatic relief of dyspnea

Contraindications
Presence of coagulopathy or hemorrhagic diathesis. If necessary, these should be corrected or minimized before procedure.

Procedure steps
Best performed with the patient sitting, leaning forward and resting arms on a bed table
- Select the drainage site by either maximum dullness to percussion (± absent or ↓ BS) or under ultrasound guidance (helpful in cases of smaller or loculated pleural effusion)
- Clean the area antiseptically and infiltrate with lidocaine 1% (25-gauge needle with 5 ml syringe). Infiltrate lidocaine into pleura. You may hear a 'pop' sound when the pleura is entered. Advance deeper, aspirate to confirm the presence of fluid
- Advance the 16 - 22 gauge needle/cannula above the rib to avoid neurovascular bundle slowly with gentle suction until fluid is aspirated. Mark the depth of the needle by applying a clamp to the needle at the skin level. Withdraw the needle and insert thoracentesis catheter and connect the cannula to 50 ml syringe and 3-way tap to drainage apparatus
- Continue to drain until no further fluid can be withdrawn, remove the needle/catheter and cover the puncture site with gauze dressing
- Obtain a CXR to evaluate fluid level and to rule out PTX

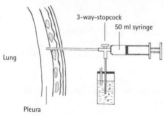

Fig. 48　Procedure for thoracocentesis

Complications

Puncture of the lung (PTX), bleeding, infection, air embolism, hypotension, spleen, intercostal artery or liver laceration

BIBLIOGRAPHY

Singer M, Webb A: Oxford Handbook of Critical Care. Oxford University Press, 1997.

Dilworth JP, Baldwin DR: Respiratory Medicine, Specialist Handbook. Martin Dunitz, 2002.

22.5　Chest Tube Drainage

Indications

Drainage of air (> 25% PTX), fluid (pleural effusion not responsive to thoracentesis), blood (hemothorax) or pus (empyema)

Steps

- Determine insertion site:
  - For PTX: anterior 2nd or 3rd intercostal space midclavicular line; direct the chest tube towards the apex of the lung
  - For pleural effusion: 5th or 6th intercostal space midaxillary line; direct the tube posteriorly
- Choose chest tube size:
  - 20 - 28 Fr for PTX, ≥ 36 Fr for fluid removal

- Prepare the area with antiseptic, anesthetize the skin and periosteum with lidocaine 1%
- Make a 2 - 3 cm skin incision over the rib to avoid neurovascular bundle which runs under the rib. Create a tunnel using hemostat to dissect and separate tissues. Inject more lidocaine into muscles and especially pleura to ease the pain
- Once the parietal pleura has been punctured, insert a gloved finger into the opening and advance the chest tube in the desired position with the hemostat or finger
- Attach the tube to a water-seal suction apparatus and apply -ve 20 cmH$_2$O suction
- Suture the tube in place with silk suture, apply occlusive dressing and secure the tubing to the chest
- Obtain CXR to check placement and assess for PTX or fluid

NOTE: Drainage tubing should not be clamped except when changing the water-seal apparatus, when the drain is elevated above the patient, during assessment if the drain can be removed and at removal.

Removal of chest tube

- Ensure resolution of PTX or hemothorax; absence of air leak on Valsava maneuver or forceful cough; < 100 ml of fluid or blood drained in 24-hour period
- Remove the tube when the pleural pressure is +ve
  - During mechanical ventilation (PPV), this occurs during inspiration
  - In a spontaneously breathing person, ask the patient to inspire fully, then perform Valsava maneuver, at which time the tube is removed rapidly
- Quickly establish an airtight seal with tape and gauzes. Obtain a follow-up CXR to document lung re-expansion

Complications

Infection, bleeding, lung laceration, subcutaneus emphysema, hemorrhage and liver or spleen injury

BIBLIOGRAPHY

Thaler DE, Hope RA, Longmore JM: Oxford Handbook of Clinical Medicine. Oxford University Press, 1999.

Dilworth JP, Baldwin DR: Respiratory Medicine, Specialist Handbook. Martin Dunitz, 2002.

22.6 Bronchoscopy

Indications

Diagnostic

- Unexplained chronic cough, hemoptysis, localized wheeze or stridor
- Suspected pulmonary infections
- Tissue sampling, staging, early diagnosis of lung cancer
- Unresolving infiltrate
- Suspected bronchopleural or tracheoesophageal (TE) fistula
- Assessment of endobronchial tube placement
- Vocal cord paralysis and hoarseness
- Assessment of airway trauma: burns, inhalational injury
- Cause of full/partial lobar or lung obstruction (e.g. blood clot, foreign body, neoplasm)
- Collection of microbiological ± cytological specimens (BAL, protected brushing, biopsy) from affected areas

Therapeutic

- Difficult intubation; double-lumen ETT; change of ETT
- Massive hemoptysis (usually with rigid bronchoscope)
- Retained secretions, mucus plugs and atelectasis
- Foreign body removal (usually with rigid bronchoscope)
- Drainage of lung abscess or bronchogenic cysts
- Fibrin glue therapy: bronchopleural fistula, PTX
- Laser, cryotherapy, brachytherapy or photodynamic therapy
- Bronchoalveolar lavage (pulmonary alveolar proteinosis)
- Stenoses and strictures (dilatation and stents)
- Directed placement of balloon catheter to arrest pulmonary bleeding

Contraindications

- Inexperienced bronchoscopist and assisting personnel
- Inadequate facilities or equipment
- Unable to adequately oxygenate the patient (severe hypoxemia)
- Patient refusal/non-compliance

- With rigid bronchoscopy: in addition to above
  - Unstable neck
  - Severely ankylosed cervical spine
  - Severe kyphoscoliosis
  - Oral or maxillofacial trauma
- Relative:
  - Acute MI or unstable ungina
  - Severe pulmonary hypertension
  - Worsening asthma
  - Coagulopathy
  - Debilitated patient

The bronchoscope: brief overview

Rigid bronchoscope:

Straight, hollow, stainless steel tube with a light source incorporated along its shaft and beveled distal end for atraumatic insertion and a variety of proximal ports. The length may be up to 40 cm, with an external diameter of up to 8 mm. The rigid bronchoscope is used much less than the fiberoptic bronchoscope (FOB) (< 5% of all bronchoscopy procedures). It is the instrument of choice for removal of foreign body and for managing massive hemoptysis because it provides a wide lumen as compared to FOB.

Fiberoptic bronchoscope:

Long, thin flexible tube that contains fibers which transmit light images. Its flexibility allows for viewing as far as subsegmental bronchi. The FOB consists of a control head unit and a soft thin shaft which contains a hollow operating channel used for suctioning, instillation of solutions or inserting instruments. The shaft is ~ 3.5 - 6 mm in external diameter (smaller for infants/children). The control unit is attached to a light source and can be fitted with a camera.

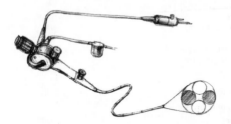

Fig. 49 Flexible fiberoptic bronchoscope with its constituent components

Procedure

- **Pre-procedure:** must get patient consent; the patient should fast overnight or feeding should be discontinued (if fed enterally) at least 6 - 8 hours prior to procedure; bronchoscopy cart and all the monitoring equipment should be in good working order
- **Premedication:** atropine is given to decrease secretions, optimize visualization, and decrease vagal reflexes; lidocaine to anesthetize upper airways; sedatives (e.g. midazolam, propofol) ± anxiolytic agent (e.g. morphine)
- Preoxygenate with 100% O_2 and monitor with pulse oximetry; if patient on ventilator, increase pressure limit alarm, increase FIO_2 to 1.0 and increase V_T by 30 - 50%. PEEP should be discontinued if possible or decreased as much as possible because airway pressures increase by as much as 25 cmH_2O during bronchoscopy. The patient should also be on AC mode. If the patient is breathing spontaneously, the venti-mask, nasal cannula or tight-fitting non-rebreather mask can be used to deliver oxygen. SpO_2 should be maintained $\geq$ 90%
- The bronchoscope is lubricated with lidocaine gel; if not intubated, lidocaine is sprayed using an atomizer (or nebulized) to the nares and pharynx
- The scope is inserted nasally or through ETT (via swivel adapter mounted on ETT to prevent loss of volume)
- Lidocaine 2% is injected into the trachea to prevent coughing and hemodynamic effects from bronchoscope stimulation of trachea and carina
- A thorough inspection and all necessary procedures are performed. If SpO_2 drops

to < 83%, the scope should be removed and the patient reoxygenated before continuing
- After the procedure, ventilator alarms and settings are reset as appropriate and a CXR ordered to exclude PTX

Risk factors/precautions
- $PaO_2 < 70$ mmHg, $FIO_2 > 0.70$
- PEEP > 10 cmH_2O or auto-PEEP > 15 cmH_2O
- Active bronchospasm
- Recent MI (< 48 h)
- Unstable arrhythmia
- MABP < 65 mmHg on vasopressors
- Coagulopathy: platelets < 20,000 - 50,000/mm^3, increased prothrombin time (PT) or partial thromboplastin time 1.5 x control
- Increased intracranial pressure

To minimize above risks
- Use ETT ≥ 8 mm internal diameter (ID) if standard scope (~ 5.5 mm diameter) is used
- Discontinue PEEP or decrease by 50%
- Use 100% O_2 starting 15 min before and during the procedure
  PaO_2 can drop by an average of 40% of baseline during the procedure
- Increase V_T by 30 - 50%
- Check ABG before and after the procedure, monitor pulse oximetry continuously $\pm$ $ETCO_2$ and BP and HR

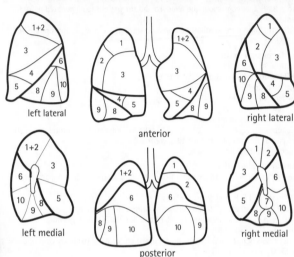

left lateral

anterior

right lateral

left medial

posterior

right medial

Left
Upper lobe
1 + 2 Apical
3 Anterior
4 Sup. segment of lingula
5 Inf. segment of lingula
Lower lobe
6 Superior
7 + 8 Ant.-med. basal
9 Lat. basal
10 Post. basal

Right
Upper lobe
1 Apical
2 Posterior
3 Anterior
Middle lobe
4 Lateral
5 Medial
Lower lobe
6 Superior
7 Med. basal 9 Lat. basal
8 Ant. basal 10 Post. basal

Fig. 50 Segments og the lungs

Ancillary procedures

Bronchial wash:

Suction port is fitted with sputum trap for wash sample. The bronchoscope is advanced to area of interest. Saline aliquots (5 - 20 ml) are injected and are immediately suctioned back. Indications: cytology and microbiology.

Bronchoalveolar wash (BAL):

The tip of the bronchoscope is wedged into a subsegmental bronchus; a known volume of saline is then injected (20 - 60 ml aliquots) and subsequently suctioned back. Up to 200 - 300 ml can be injected. It may be diagnostic in pulmonary hemorrhage, eosinophilic pneumonia, alveolar proteinosis, differentiating interstitial lung disease (e.g. sarcoidosis, hypersensitivity pneumonitis), ARDS, malignancy.

Bronchial brushing:

A soft brush is inserted through the working channel of the bronchoscope into the area of interest. Cells are collected by brushing up and down the airway. The brush is then retracted into the sheath and the sheathed brush is removed from the bronchoscope. Used for cytological studies.

Protected bronchial brushing:

The protected brush is advanced to the site of the lesion and a biodegradable plug is dislodged. The inner catheter is advanced and the brush is moved forward into the distal airways. After collecting the specimen, the brush is withdrawn into the inner catheter and the entire apparatus is extracted (must remove and process brush using sterile technique). Protected bronchial brushing is used for bacteriology, when need to collect samples that reflect bacteria of lower airways rather than upper airways.

Bronchial biopsy:

Biopsy forceps are advanced to the area of interest and forceps are opened and closed firmly to sample the lesion. Used for sampling visible abnormal lesions.
A mass that is too deep within the lung tissue (periphery) requires a biopsy using fluoroscopic guidance.

Transbronchial lung biopsy:

Biopsy under fluoroscopic guidance. Helpful in interstitial lung disease, peripheral nodules and diffuse infective lung disease.

Transbronchial needle aspiration:

Sheathed needle is passed through the working channel of bronchoscope and is then advanced through tracheal or carinal wall and aspirated. The needle is withdrawn into the sheath, the sheath is extracted and then a sample is placed on a slide for analysis under a microscope. Procedure is indicated for diagnosis and staging of bronchogenic carcinoma, diagnosis of peribronchial/tracheal masses and peripheral lung nodules.

Possible complications
- Fever and flu-like symptoms (usually resolve in < 24 h)
- Related to medications:
  - Oversedation ⇒ decreased respiratory drive, hypoventilation, hypoxemia, hypercapnia, syncope
  - Lidocaine toxicity ⇒ seizures, convulsions, bradycardia, hypotension, bronchospasm
- Trauma (with rigid bronchoscopy): damage to dentures, soft tissue, vocal cords
- PTX: usually only with biopsy or brushing
- Hypoxemia, arrhythmias, hemorrhage

BIBLIOGRAPHY

Tai DYH: Bronchoscopy in the Intensive Care Unit. Ann Acad Med Singapore 1998; 27: 552-559.

Raoof S, Mehrishi S, Prakash UB: Role of Bronchoscopy in Modern Medical Intensive Care Unit. Clin Chest Med 2001; 22: 241-261.

Sachs S: Fiberoptic Bronchoscopy. In, Hess DR et al (eds): Respiratory Care: Principles and Practice. WB Saunders, 2002.

Singer M, Webb A: Oxford Handbook of Critical Care. Oxford University Press, 1997.

Dilworth JP, Baldwin DR: Respiratory Medicine, Specialist Handbook. Martin Dunitz, 2002.

22.7 Intubation

Indications

- To prevent aspiration resulting from inadequate upper airway reflexes
- To facilitate suctioning: excessive secretions, ↓/absent cough
- To relieve airway obstruction
- Need for mechanical ventilation

> **NOTE:** If the patient is expected to require an artificial airway for > 15 - 21 days, a tracheostomy tube (TT) may be preferred.

Equipment

- **ETT of various sizes;** minimal: 7 mm ID for most **females** and 8 - 9 mm ID for most **males**
- **10 ml syringe:** attached to balloon port of ETT
- **Lubricant:** lubricate stylet before inserting into ETT and lubricate bottom ¼ of ETT
- **Stylet:** to make ETT more rigid; make sure that distal end is not protruding through the end of ETT (bend it at proximal end of ETT so it is ~ 1 cm away from the distal end of ETT); NOT for nasotracheal intubation
- **Bag and mask:** connected to O_2 source
- **Oral, nasal airways:** various sizes
- **Suction:** catheters, tonsillar (Yankauer) tip
- **Tape** (cloth) or other method for securing tube
- **Laryngoscope(s):** straight (Miller), curved (Macintosh): check light bulbs, extra batteries

Adult:	No. 3 or 4 curved blade
Child < 8 years	No. 2 curved blade
Term infant	No. 1 straight blade
Premature baby	No. 0 straight blade

- **Monitoring:** pulse ox, EKG, BP, $EtCO_2$ detector, stethoscope
- **Medication:** sedatives, NM blockers and reversals may be needed

Procedure

- **Position patient** supine and flex head back to achieve 'sniffing position'; may place folded towel or pillow under head; *neck trauma:* neutral position

- **Preoxygenate** with 100% O_2 via bag and mask for > 3 - 5 min to ↑ O_2 reserve (washes out N_2, allowing more time before SaO_2 ↓ to < 90%)
- Assistant may **apply cricoid pressure** (compresses esophagus) to ↓ risk of aspiration of gastric contents
- **Open mouth** with right hand and with left hand **insert blade** into right side of mouth
- Elevate tongue and move it to the left
- **Advance** tip of **blade** into the vallecula (curved blade) or under the epiglottis (straight blade)

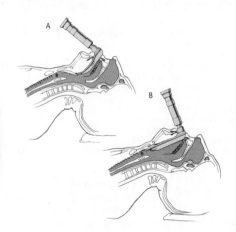

Fig. 51 The curved blade (left) is inserted into the vallecula, while the straight blade directly lifts the epiglottis (right)

- Gently **lift blade** upward; glottis should now be visible (vocal cords)
- **Pass ETT through vocal cords** (cuff 1 - 2 cm below); usually ETT is advanced until the mark reaches the teeth (a distance of ~ 21 cm for F and ~ 23 cm for M); (pull out stylet if used)

NOTE: *Intubation attempt should not last > 30 seconds (20 s in newborns) and between attempts patient should be hyperoxygenated with BMV. If the intubationist is unable to successfully intubate in 2 - 3 attempts, another clinician should give it a try.*

NOTE: *Drugs that can be administered down the ETT include lidocaine, atropine, naloxone and epinephrine (LANE). The dose of these medications is usually 2½ x its usual dose, added in 5 - 10 ml of normal saline.*

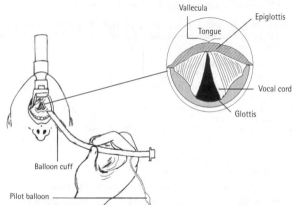

Fig. 52 The tongue is pushed leftward with the blade, the vocal cords are visualized and the endotracheal tube is inserted. Pilot balloon is used to inflate the ETT balloon cuff with a 5 ml or 10 ml syringe

Fig. 53 Cross-section of the glottis

Postintubation

- **Inflate cuff** just enough to seal air leak
- **Confirm placement:** while bagging, check for +ve and equal bilateral breath sounds at axilla, (+ve bilateral chest rise) and listen over the epigastrium for any gurgling sounds; if heard = esophageal intubation ⇒ withdraw tube, oxygenate and reattempt with new ETT
- If BS diminished/absent on left side, most likely = right mainstem intubation: deflate cuff, pull out ETT 1 - 2 cm and listen for bilateral BS
- May also confirm proper placement with disposable ET-CO_2 detector:
  - No CO_2 = ETT probably in esophagus (no color change)
  - ETT in trachea = device changes color from purple to yellow

> ***NOTE 1:*** *May be falsely negative in cardiac arrest (no CO_2 returning to lungs).*
> ***NOTE 2:*** *Newer models of resuscitation bags have ET-CO_2 detector included as one of its components.*

Other confirmation methods

- Condensation 'fog' of ETT during mechanical ventilation = unreliable
- Aspirator bulb: attached while compressed to ETT and released: bulb reexpands = ETT in trachea; No reexpansion = esophageal intubation
- Once sure tube is in trachea, secure it with tape or other type of holder, preferably to upper jaw, as it does not move compared with lower jaw
- Attempt to keep $P_{cuff} < 25 - 35$ cmH$_2$O (18 - 25 mmHg) to ↓ risk of pressure necrosis/ischemia to trachea; P_{cuff} too low = aspiration risk; appropriate pressure depends upon size of ETT (smaller needs higher pressure and may be replaced with larger), size of ID of trachea and shape of trachea
- Finally, **obtain CXR** to confirm

Guide to choosing ETT sizes, suction catheter and laryngoscope blade

Age/weight	ETT ID (mm)	Distance of Insertion (cm)	Suction catheter (Fr)	Laryngoscope blade
< 1 kg	2.5 **U**	7	5 - 6	Straight (0)
1 - 2 kg	3.0 **N**	8	6 - 8	
2 - 3 kg	3.5 **C**	9		
> 3 kg - 6 mo	3.5 **U**	10		Straight (1)
1 year	4.0 **F**	11		

3 year	4.5	F	12 – 13	8	Curved (2)
5 year	5	E	> 2 years = age in years/2 +12 cm	10	
8 year	6	D			
10 – 12 years	6.5			12	
12 – 16 years	7				Curved (3)
Adult female	7 - 8		21		
Adult male	8 - 9		23		

NOTE: ETT with 8 yo = uncuffed; French (Fr) size = ID/2) x 3
Straight = Miller blade; Curved = MacIntosh blade.

22.8   Extubation

- Have patient in semi-Fowler's position and explain procedure
- Preoxygenate patient for $\geq$ 1 min (by BMV if necessary)
- Suction trachea and oropharynx
- Deflate cuff and untape ETT
- Ask patient to take deep breath and withdraw ETT at end-inspiration
- Ask patient to cough to clear secretions
- Give O_2 $\pm$ cool aerosol; may $\uparrow$ FIO_2 by ~10% > FIO_2 on ventilator
- Monitor patient for dyspnea, stridor, obstruction and encourage deep breaths and cough
- Stridor resulting from glottic $\pm$ subglottic edema is treated with cool aerosol and 0.5 ml of 2.25% **racemic epinephrine** in 5 ml normal saline to $\downarrow$ swelling; **Dexamethasone?**

Removal of the endotracheal tube (ETT)

Setting:
ETT should be removed in an environment in which the patient can be monitored and emergency equipment and appropriately trained staff with airway care skills are immediately available.

Indications:
- Airway control no longer needed
- Artificial airway obstruction (unable to clear rapidly, e.g. massive mucus plug)
- Discontinuance if further medical care is needed

Contraindications:
- No absolute

Hazards/complications:
- Hypoxemia
- Hypercapnia
- Death

Assessment of the need:
- Artificial airway no longer needed as indicated by:
  - Adequate spontaneous ventilation and ability to meet weaning criteria:
    - Adequate PaO_2 on PEEP < 10 cmH$_2$O, FIO$_2$ < 0.4
    - Maintain appropriate pH and $PaCO_2$
    - C_{thorax} (thoracic compliance) > 25 ml/cmH$_2$O
    - RR < 35/min
    - MIP > 30 cmH$_2$O
    - MVV > 2 x resting V_E
    - RR/V_T ≤ 98 - 130
    - V_C > 10 ml/kg IBW
    - V_D/V_T < 0.6
    - V_E (spontaneous) < 10 L/min

Resolution of need for airway protection:
- Normal consciousness
- Adequate airway protection reflexes
- Easily managed secretions

Assessment of outcome/monitoring:
- Assess/monitor
- Spontaneous ventilation
- ABGs (invasive, non-invasive)
- Chest X-ray
- Complications
- Need for reintubation

From AARC Clinical Practice Guideline: Removal of the Endotracheal Tube, Respir Care 1999; vol 44, No 1: 85-90

22.9   Suctioning

Indications: as needed (prn)
- Gurgling, noisy breathing (rhonchi)
- Visible secretions in the oropharynx or ETT
- To obtain a sputum specimen
- ↑ PIP with volume ventilation or ↓ V_T with pressure ventilation
- Inability to cough effectively as a result of coma or NM disease

Technique: sterile
- **Preoxygenate** patient with 100% O_2 (for neonates, use 10% higher FIO_2 than being used at the time -100% if necessary, e.g. PPHN)
- Gently insert catheter without vacuum until obstruction is felt (carina), pull back 1 cm and apply intermittent suction while removing catheter (whole procedure should take < 10 s)
- Recommended -ve pressure:
  Infant/child ~ 40 – 80 mmHg, adult ~ 100 – 140 mmHg
- May instill a few ml of normal saline to liquefy thick secretions and stimulate cough; this may dislodge bacteria from ETT into lower airways and should not be used routinely
- **Reoxygenate** patient with 100% O_2 and repeat suction if needed

Complications
- **Airway trauma** due to high (-ve) pressures used or 'rough' technique
- **Hypoxemia** due to inappropriate long suction time or no preoxygenation
- **Hypotension** due to bradycardia (vagal stimulation)
- Discomfort, pain, **bronchospasm**, coughing, ↑ICP
- **Atelectasis** due to a too long suction time, a too high vacuum pressure or a too wide suction catheter (this may be avoided by using a catheter that is < ½ ID of artificial airway)
- **Arrhythmias:** Premature ventricular complexes (myocardium hypoxia); **bradycardia (vagal stimulation)**, tachycardia (from hypoxemia, pain or anxiety)

22.10 Cricothyroidotomy

Indications

Upper airway obstruction when intubation is not possible (e.g. irretrievable foreign body, facial trauma). It is a temporary intervention, until a more formal airway can be established. Allows oxygenation, but CO_2 is not eliminated, therefore, it is only useful for about 30–45 min.

Procedure

Needle cricothyroidotomy:

- With the patient in a supine position, palpate the cricothyroid membrane between the thyroid and cricoid cartilages
- Insert a 14 G catheter attached to a saline filled syringe through the cricothyroid membrane, directed caudally, then aspirate with the syringe Air will enter the syringe when the needle enters the trachea
- Slide the catheter into the trachea and remove the needle
- Deliver oxygen: various adapters can be used to attach to the catheter, e.g.
  (1) tracheostomy collar with spontaneously breathing patient
  (2) resuscitation bag (connect 3 ml syringe to the needle, then use 15 mm adapter from a 7.5 mm ID ETT to which resuscitation bag is attached
  (3) Y-connector placed in the catheter and connected to O_2 tubing, with the open end of the Y occluded for 1 second out of 5 seconds to allow O_2 to enter
  (4) connect 10 ml syringe to catheter and insert 7 mm ID ETT into syringe, then inflate the cuff to create seal. Other connectors may be used

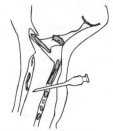

Fig. 54 Needle cricothyroidotomy

Surgical cricothyroidotomy:
- The cricothyroid membrane is localized, local anesthetic is infiltrated if necessary and a transverse incision of 2 - 3 cm is made through the skin and then the membrane. A scalpel with No. 11 blade is ideal, but any sharp instrument may be used if a scalpel is not available, such as pocket knife, scissors, large bore needle
- The hole can be dilated if necessary by using a hemostat or simply inserting and rotating the scalpel handle by 90°
- A tracheostomy tube or ETT (cut short) is inserted, the cuff is inflated and the tube is secured in place
- This procedure is not recommended in children < 12 - 13 years of age

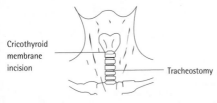

Cricothyroid membrane incision

Tracheostomy

Fig. 55 Surgical cricothyroidotomy

Complications
- Creation of false passage
- Posterior laceration of trachea/esophagus
- Bleeding, infection, barotraumas (subcutaneous emphysema)
- Possible stenosis; surgical cricothyroidotomy should be converted to tracheostomy electively within 24 hours
- Kinking, breakage or dislodgement of the needle/catheter

BIBLIOGRAPHY

Finucane BT, Santora AH: Principles of Airway Management, 3rd ed. Springer-Verlag, 2003.

Hanowell LH, Waldron RJ: Airway Management. Lippincott-Raven, 1996.

Müller S: Memorix: Emergency Medicine. Chapman & Hall Medical, 1997.

22.11 Tracheostomy

Indications
- To relieve upper airway obstruction
- To provide a means for ventilatory support
- For relief of obstructive sleep apnea
- Pulmonary toilet
- Prophylaxis: extensive head/neck procedures

Contraindications
- Uncorrectable bleeding diatheses: PT or activated thromboplastin time > 1.5 x and platelets < 50,000/μL
- Neck distortion
- Tracheomalacia
- < 13 - 15-year-olds
- Prior major neck surgery

Advantages over intubation
- Eases airway care, tube reinsertion and suctioning
- Decreased risk for extubation
- Decreased risk for upper airway complications related to ETT
- Facilitates communication and speech
- Improves comfort, hygiene and patient appearance and mobility

Procedure: only **percutaneous dilatational tracheostomy (PDT)** is described
- The patient is positioned with the neck extended and the skin of the area of puncture is infiltrated with lidocaine 2% and epinephrine 1/100,000
- Before the incision is made, the ETT cuff is deflated and the tip of the tube withdrawn to the level of the cricoid cartilage
- A small incision is made between the 2nd and 3rd tracheal rings and a 14 G cannula is inserted into the trachea between the 1st and 2nd tracheal rings
- A guidewire is introduced through the cannula under direct bronchoscopic vision and the stoma is dilated with increasing sizes of plastic dilators
- A lubricated tracheostomy tube loaded over an appropriately sized dilator (e.g. 21 Fr dilator for 7 mm ID tracheostomy tube) is introduced into trachea and the guidewire plus dilator are removed
- The cuff is inflated and the tube secured with tracheostomy tube Velcro holder (or cloth ties). If indicated, the ventilator is connected to the tracheostomy tube
- The ETT is removed after confirming correct tracheostomy tube position (e.g. bronchoscopy, auscultation)

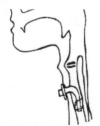

Fig. 56 Tracheostomy tube in place

Complications

- Bleeding
- False channel insertion
- Posterior trachea or esophagus laceration
- Stenosis
- Tracheitis
- Tracheomalacia
- Tracheoesophageal fistula
- Granulation
- Scarring
- Postobstructive pulmonary edema
- Barotraumas (e.g. PTX, subcutaneous emphysema)
- Stomal infection
- Tube obstruction/dislodgement
- Vocal cord dysfunction

Types of tracheostomy tube

Standard cuffed tracheostomy tube:

Available in sizes 2.5 - 11.5 mm ID. There are different shapes available: curved, angled, extra long distally (e.g. when it is necessary to bypass an obstruction in the trachea) or extra long proximally (e.g. patient with obese neck). The removable inner cannula has a standard 15 mm adapter, which provides a point of attachment for other respiratory equipment (e.g. ventilator circuit). An obturator with a rounded tip (to prevent trauma) is used for (re)insertion of the tracheostomy tube through the stoma. Should be kept at patient's bedside in case the patient decannulates.

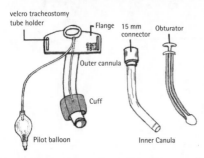

Fig. 57 Typical cuffed tracheostomy tube. Disposable inner cannula is replaced daily and the obturator is used for (re)insertion of tracheostomy tube; its rounded end is designed for atraumatic insertion of tracheostomy tube

Uncuffed tracheostomy tubes:

These are used mainly in (1) pediatric patients because of small trachea and narrow cricoid ring and (2) as a method of weaning from tracheostomy tube. Progressively smaller diameters of uncuffed tubes are used to allow suctioning and maintenance of stoma while allowing the patient to adapt to normal airway.

Fenestrated:

Useful when need to assess patient readiness to be decannulated and for allowing the patient to talk when the tube is occluded with a plug (with removed inner cannula and deflated cuff). This allows the patient to inhale and exhale through the fenestration and around the tube. The problem with this tube is that the fenestrations are rarely in the correct place (e.g. against the posterior trachea ⇒ obstruction and tissue growth into fenestrations). Simply deflating the cuff or downsizing to a cuffless tube may be preferred over fenestrated tube.

Talking tracheostomy tubes:

Rarely used, as other, more convenient devices are available (e.g. Passy-Muir speaking valve, see below). This tube has an opening in the posterior portion of the cuff, through which a source of gas is provided for speech. The patient occludes the open end of the Y connector when they need to phonate.

Other devices

Tracheal button:

Rarely used; for temporary maintenance of tracheostomy stoma, e.g. when need to change tracheostomy tube at a later date or for suctioning. Consists of a hollow outer cannula and inner solid cannula, which fits from the skin to just inside the anterior wall of the trachea.

Passy – Muir tracheostomy speaking valve:

This one-way valve is attached to a 15 mm universal adapter of the tracheostomy tube with the cuff deflated. It opens on inspiration and closes on expiration; this directs exhaled air to pass through the vocal cords, permitting speech. These devices can be used in spontaneously breathing or mechanically ventilated patients.

NOTE: *Use with caution in patients at risk of aspiration because the tracheostomy tube cuff must be deflated. If used during mechanical ventilation, may need to increase V_T to compensate for leakage and lost volume around deflated cuff; it should be used with AC mode of ventilation, as modes such as PS cannot be used with deflated cuffs.*

BIBLIOGRAPHY

Finucane BT, Santora AH: Principles of Airway Management, 3rd ed. Springer Verlag 2003.

May AR, Bortner LP: Airway Management. In, Hess DR, et al: Respiratory Care: Principles and Practice. WB Saunders, 2002.

Simmons KF, Scanlan CL: Airway Management. In, Wilkins RL, Stoller JK, Scanlan CL (eds): Egan's Fundamentals of Respiratory Care, 8th ed. Elsevier Science Limited, 2003.

APPENDICES

23. Appendix 1

23.1 Abbreviations/Symbols

NOTE: *Some of the following abbreviations and symbols are used more often than others throughout the text, while some which have been used infrequently - or not at all - are included for the sake of completeness, as they may be used/seen in medical charting. Check your facility's policy (if any) for approved abbreviations and/or symbols.*

Symbols

°:	degree
? :	unknown, questionable
=:	equals
≈:	equals approximately
≠:	not equal to
~:	about
# or No:	number
±:	plus or minus; with or without
x:	multiplied by; times
÷ or /:	divided by
>:	greater than
>>:	much greater than
<:	less than
<<:	much less than
≥:	greater than or equal to
≤:	less than or equal to
↑:	increase
↑↑, ↑:	large increase
↓:	decrease
↓↓, ↓:	large decrease
⇒:	leads to; results in
1°:	primarily due to

2°:	secondary to
3°:	tertiary, 3rd degree
M:	male
F:	female

Abbreviations

A

AARC:	American Association of Respiratory Care
ATS:	American Thoracic Society
ABG:	arterial blood gases
AE:	adverse effects
AC:	assist control
ac:	before meals
ARDS:	adult respiratory distress syndrome
ALS:	amyotrophic lateral sclerosis
A-C:	alveolar capillary
Ach:	acetylcholine
AMBU:	air mask bag unit
A-P:	anteroposterior
A1AT:	alpha 1 antitrypsin
ASAP:	as soon as possible
aka:	also known as
ant:	anterior
ASD:	atrial septal defect
a-v:	arterio-venous
atm:	atmosphere
ANS:	autonomic nervous system
AIDS:	acquired immune deficiency syndrome

B

BP:	blood pressure
BD:	bronchodilator
bid:	twice daily
BPD:	bronchopulmonary dysplasia
BUN:	blood urea nitrogen

b/l:	bilateral
bpm:	beats or breaths per minute
BMV:	bag mask ventilator
BSA:	body surface area

C

°C:	degree Celsius
COPD:	chronic obstructive pulmonary disease
CO:	cardiac output or carbon monoxide
CO_2:	carbon dioxide
C:	compliance
C_L:	lung compliance
C_{st}:	static compliance
C_{dyn}:	dynamic compliance
CHF:	congestive heart failure
CVP:	central venous pressure
CPR:	cardiopulmonary resuscitation
CI:	cardiac index or contraindications
CSF:	cerebrospinal fluid
CT:	computed tomography
CSA:	central sleep apnea
CBC:	complete blood count
CXR:	chest X-ray
cm:	centimeter
CV:	cardiovascular
cmH_2O:	centimeters of water
CF:	cystic fibrosis
CDH:	congenital diaphragmatic hernia
C&S:	culture and sensitivity
COHb:	carboxyhemoglobin
CPAP:	constant positive airway pressure
CaO_2:	arterial oxygen content
CvO_2:	mixed venous oxygen content
c/o:	complains of
CC:	chief complaint

CS:	corticosteroids
CA:	cancer
CAD:	coronary artery disease
CW:	chest wall

D

d:	day
DVT:	deep vein thrombosis
DPI:	dry powder inhaler
DKA:	diabetic ketoacidosis
dl:	deciliter
DOE:	dyspnea on exertion
D_LCO:	carbon monoxide diffusing capacity
DO_2:	oxygen delivery
dc:	discontinue
DNR:	do not resuscitate
DNI:	do not intubate
Dx:	diagnosis
Dz:	disease

E

$ETCO_2$:	end-tidal exhaled carbon dioxide
EF:	effects
EKG or ECG:	electrocardiogram
ETT:	endotracheal tube
ECMO:	extracorporeal membrane oxygenation
EPAP:	expiratory positive airway pressure
ENT:	ears, nose and throat
EENT:	eyes, ears, nose and throat
EEG:	electroencephalogram
ERS:	European Respiratory Society
ESR:	erythrocyte sedimentation rate

F

°F:	degree Fahrenheit
ft:	foot
FRC:	functional residual capacity
FIO_2:	fraction of inspired oxygen
FVC:	forced vital capacity
FEV_1:	forced expiratory volume in one second
FR:	flow rate
FHR:	fetal heart rate
fv:	fever
fx:	fracture(s)

G

GI:	gastrointestinal
GERD:	gastro-esophageal reflux disease
GCS:	Glasgow Coma Scale
GFR:	glomerular filtration rate
GYN:	gynecology

H

h or hr:	hour
hs:	hours of sleep
HEENT:	head, eyes, ears, nose and throat
Hb:	hemoglobin
HR:	heart rate
Hx:	history
HTN:	hypertension
Ht:	height
Hct:	hematocrit
HFV:	high frequency ventilation
HCO_3^-:	bicarbonate
H_2O:	water
HOB:	head of bed
HMD:	hyaline membrane disease
HME:	heat moisture exchanger

HIV:	human immunodeficiency virus

I

IVC:	inferior vena cava
IRDS:	infant respiratory distress syndrome
ICP:	intracranial pressure
IV:	intravenous
IM:	intramuscular
Infx:	infection(s)
IBW:	ideal body weight
I&O:	input and output
ICU:	intensive care unit
IPPV:	invasive positive pressure ventilation

J

JVD:	jugular venous distension

K

K:	potassium
KCl:	potassium chloride
kg:	kilogram

L

L:	liter
LBW:	low birth weight
LA:	left atrium
LHF:	left heart failure
lb:	pound
LRTI:	lower respiratory tract infection

M

MV:	mechanical ventilation
MA:	mechanism or mode of action
m:	meter
Mg^{++}:	magnesium

mo:	month
MAS:	meconium aspiration syndrome
MI:	myocardial infarction
MIP:	maximum inspiratory pressure
MAP or	
MAWP:	mean airway pressure
Maint:	maintenance
MABP:	mean arterial blood pressure
MG:	myasthenia gravis
metHb:	methemoglobin

N

NO:	nitric oxide
NICU:	neonatal intensive care unit
NB:	newborn
NPPV:	non-invasive positive pressure ventilation
NM:	neuromuscular
NC:	nasal cannula
NS:	normal saline
NG:	nasogastric
NPO:	nothing by mouth
NKA:	no known allergies
N_2:	nitrogen

O

O_2:	oxygen
OSA:	obstructive sleep apnea
OD:	overdose

P

P_{aw}:	airway pressure
P:	pressure
PA:	pulmonary artery
Pb:	barometric pressure
PIP:	peak inspiratory pressure or peak pressure (P_{peak})

prn:	as needed
PO:	by mouth
PSV:	pressure support ventilation
PPHN:	persistent pulmonary hypertension of newborn
PDA:	patent ductus arteriosus
Ped:	pediatric
pc:	after meals
PEEP:	positive end-expiratory pressure
PAWP:	pulmonary artery wedge pressure
PPV:	positive pressure ventilation
PVC:	premature ventricular contractions
P_{alv}:	alveolar pressure
PaO_2:	arterial oxygen tension
PAO_2:	alveolar oxygen tension
$PaCO_2$:	arterial carbon dioxide tension
$PACO_2$:	alveolar carbon dioxide tension
PRVC:	pressure regulated volume control
PND:	paroxysmal nocturnal dyspnea
PC:	pressure control
PLV:	partial liquid ventilation
PE:	pulmonary embolism
Pt:	patient
PTX:	pneumothorax
P_{ven}:	pulmonary venous pressure

Q

Q:	every
qd:	every day
qid:	4 times daily

R

Rx:	treatment
r/o:	rule out
R_{aw}:	airway resistance
RBC:	red blood cell

Rt:	right
RR:	respiratory rate
RLD:	restrictive lung disease
RV:	right ventricle
RHF:	right heart failure

S

SVC:	superior vena cava
SVR:	systemic vascular resistance
SOB:	shortness of breath
SaO_2:	arterial oxygen saturation
SIMV:	synchronized intermittent mandatory ventilation
Sz:	seizure
s/sx:	signs and symptoms
SC:	subcutaneous

T

T:	temperature
TOF:	tetralogy of Fallot
TT:	tracheostomy tube
Tid:	3 times per day
TB:	tuberculosis
Tx:	treatment
Torr:	partial pressure equivalent to mmHg
Ti:	inspiratory time
Te:	expiratory time
TTN:	transient tachypnea of the newborn

U

URTI:	upper respiratory tract infection
UTI:	urinary tract infection
UAO:	upper airway obstruction

V

$V_A P$:	ventilator associated pneumonia
V_C:	vital capacity
V_D/V_T:	dead space to tidal volume ratio
V_A:	alveolar volume
VCO_2:	carbon dioxide production
VO_2:	oxygen consumption
V_E:	minute ventilation
V_D:	dead space
V_T:	tidal volume
VLBW:	very low birth weight
VCD:	vocal cord dysfunction

W

WOB:	work of breathing
wk:	week
WBC:	white blood cells
wt:	weight
WNL:	within normal limits
w/o:	without

Y

yr or y:	year
yo:	year old

24.   Appendix 2

24.1   Equations

24.1.1   Oxygenation

Alveolar oxygen tension (PAO$_2$)
$P_AO_2 = (Pb - PH_2O) \times FIO_2 - (PaCO_2 \times 1.25)$
Normal: 100 mmHg room air and 673 mmHg on 100% O_2

Alveolar to arterial oxygen tension (A - a) gradient or P(A - a)O$_2$
$= P_AO_2 - PaO_2$
Normal: 5 - 20 mmHg room air and 25 - 65 mmHg on 100% O_2
Increased: V/Q mismatch, R - L shunt, diffusion defect

P/F (oxygenation ratio)
$= PaO_2/FIO_2$
Normal: > 200, regardless of FIO_2

Arterial oxygen content (CaO$_2$)
$CaO_2 = (Hb \times 1.34 \times SaO_2) + (PaO_2 \times 0.003)$
Normal: 18 - 21 ml/dl

Mixed venous oxygen content (CvO$_2$)
$CvO_2 = (Hb \times 1.34 \times SvO_2) + (PvO_2 \times 0.003)$
Normal: 12 - 15 ml/dl

Arterial - venous oxygen content difference (C(a - v)O$_2$)
$C(a-v)O_2 = CaO_2 - CvO_2$
Normal: 4 - 5 ml/dl; O_2 consumed by tissues

Oxygen consumption (VO$_2$)
$VO_2 = CO \times C(a - v)O_2 \times 10$
Normal: ~ 250 ml/min

Respiratory quotient (RQ)
VCO_2/VO_2 ratio at tissue level; (internal respiration)
Normal: 0.8 - 0.85; glucose = 1.0; protein = 0.8; fat = 0.7

RER (respiratory exchange ratio): VCO_2/VO_2 ratio in lungs; external respiration
Normal: $VCO_2/VO_2 = 200/250 = 0.8$
RQ $\approx$ RER at steady state

Oxygen delivery (DO_2)
$DO_2 = (CO \times CaO_2) \times 10$
Normal: 750 - 1000 ml/min

Oxygen extraction ratio (O_2ER)
$O_2ER = (CaO_2 - CvO_2) / CaO_2$
Normal: 25%

24.1.2 Ventilation

Minute ventilation (V_E)
$VE = V_T \times RR$
Normal: 5 - 8 L/min

Alveolar ventilation (V_A)
$V_A = VE - V_D$ (for 1 min)
Normal: $\frac{2}{3}$ of VE
$V_A = V_T - V_D$ (for 1 breath)
Normal: $\frac{2}{3}$ of V_T

Dead space ventilation (V_D)
$V_D = V_Dphys \times RR$
$V_D = V_E - V_A$
Normal: $\frac{1}{3}$ of V_E; estimated V_Danat = 1 ml/lb or 2ml/kg IBW or 0.5 ml/lb intubated

Dead space to tidal volume ratio (V_D/V_T)
$V_D/V_T = (PaCO_2 - PECO_2)/PaCO_2$
Normal: 0.25 - 0.35

24.1.3 Hemodynamics

Cardiac output (CO)
$CO = SV \times HR$
$CO = VO_2 \div (CaO_2 - CvO_2) \times 10$
Normal: 4 - 8 L/min

Cardiac index (CI)
CI = CO/BSA
Normal: 2.5 - 4.5 L/min/m^2

Mean arterial blood pressure (MABP)
MABP = (2 x diaBP + sysBP)/3
Normal: 80 - 100 mmHg

Stroke volume (SV)
SV = CO/HR
Normal: 60 - 120 ml/beat

Pulmonary vascular resistance (PVR)
PVR = 80 x (meanPAP - PAWP)/3
Normal: < 200 dynes x s x cm^{-5}

Systemic vascular resistance (SVR)
SVR = 80 x (MABP - CVP)/CO
Normal: 900 - 1600 dynes x s x cm^{-5}

24.1.4   Ventilator

Static compliance (C_{st})
$C_{st} = V_T / (P_{plat} - PEEP)$
Normal: > 60 ml/cmH$_2$O

Dynamic compliance (C_{dyn})
$C_{dyn} = V_T / (PIP - PEEP)$
Normal: 40 ml/cmH$_2$O

Airway resistance (R_{aw})
$R_{aw} = (PIP - P_{plat}) \div$ flow (in L/sec)
Normal: 0.5 - 2.5; intubated ~ 5 - 8 cmH$_2$O/L/s

24.1.5   Miscellanous

Ideal body weight (IBW)
Male: 50 kg + (2.3 kg per inch over 5 ft)
Female: 45 kg + (2.3 kg per inch over 5 ft)

Body surface area (BSA)
BSA in m^2 = (Ht in cm x 0.725) x (Wt in kg x 0.425) x 0.007145

25. Appendix 3

25.1 Conversions

Temperature
°C = (°F - 32) x 1.8
°F = (°C x 1.8) + 32
Normal: 37 °C (98.6 °F)
Normal range: 36.5 - 37.5 °C
Freezing point: 0 °C or 32 °F
Interesting fact: - 40 °C = - 40 °F

Weight
kg = lb x 0.454 (1 lb = 454 g)
lb = kg x 2.2 (1 kg = 2.2 lb)
1 oz = 28 g

Distance
1 in = 2.54 cm
1 cm = 0.39 in
1 m = 100 cm = 1000 mm
1 m = 39.37 in = 1.09 yards
1 km = 1000 m = 0.62 mile
1 ft = 30.48 cm = 12 in
1 mile = 1.61 km

Pressure
1 mmHg = 1.36 cmH$_2$O
1 cmH$_2$O = 0.735 mmHg
760 mmHg = 1 atmosphere

Volume
1 L = 1000 ml
1 L = 1.06 qt
1 gallon = 3.785 L
1 tsp = 5 ml
1 tbs = 15 ml

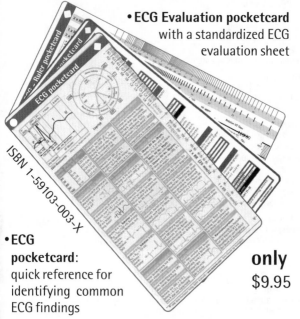

Index

italic= tradename, **bold** = drug

B

D

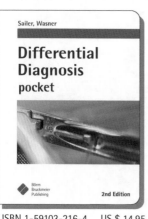

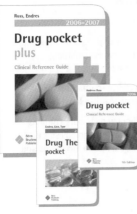

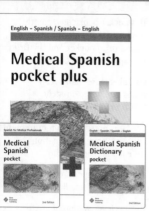

Börm Bruckmeier Publishing
PO Box 388
Ashland, OH 44805

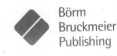

Börm
Bruckmeier
Publishing

Phone: 888-322-6657
Fax: 419-281-6883

Name		E-mail	
Address			
City		State	Zip

		Subtotal	
Sales Tax, add only for: CA 8%; OH 6.25%		+ Sales Tax	
Shipping & Handling for US address:		+ S&H	
UPS Standard: 1 0% of subtotal with a minimum of $5.00			
UPS 2nd Day Air: 20% of subtotal with a minimum of $8.00			
		= Total	

Credit Card: ☐ Visa ☐ Mastercard ☐ Amex ☐ Discover
Card Number

Exp. Date   Signature

**For foreign orders,
quantity rebate, optional
shipping and payment
please inquire:
service@media4u.com**

Books and Pocketcards also available at...

www. media4u .com

Börm Bruckmeier Products

	COPIES		PRICE/COPIES		PRICE
pockets					
Anatomy pocket		x	US $ 16.95	=	
Canadian Drug pocket 2006–2007		x	US $ 14.95	=	
Differential Diagnosis pocket		x	US $ 14.95	=	
Drug pocket 2006		x	US $ 12.95	=	
Drug pocket plus 2006–2007		x	US $ 24.95	=	
Drug Therapy pocket 2006–2007		x	US $ 16.95	=	
ECG pocket		x	US $ 16.95	=	
ECG Cases pocket		x	US $ 16.95	=	
EMS pocket		x	US $ 14.95	=	
Homeopathy pocket		x	US $ 14.95	=	
Medical Abbreviations pocket		x	US $ 16.95	=	
Medical Classifications pocket		x	US $ 16.95	=	
Medical Spanish pocket		x	US $ 16.95	=	
Medical Spanish Dictionary pocket		x	US $ 16.95	=	
Medical Spanish pocket plus		x	US $ 22.95	=	
Normal Values pocket		x	US $ 12.95	=	
Respiratory pocket		x	US $ 16.95	=	
pocketcards					
Alcohol Withdrawal pocketcard		x	US $ 3.95	=	
Antibiotics pocketcard 2006		x	US $ 3.95	=	
Antifungals pocketcard		x	US $ 3.95	=	
ECG pocketcard		x	US $ 3.95	=	
ECG Evaluation pocketcard		x	US $ 3.95	=	
ECG Ruler pocketcard		x	US $ 3.95	=	
ECG pocketcard Set (3)		x	US $ 9.95	=	
Echocardiography pocketcard Set (2)		x	US $ 6.95	=	
H&P pocketcard		x	US $ 3.95	=	
Medical Abbreviations pocketcard Set (2)		x	US $ 6.95	=	
Medical Spanish pocketcard		x	US $ 3.95	=	
Medical Spanish pocketcard Set (2)		x	US $ 6.95	=	
Neurology pocketcard Set (2)		x	US $ 6.95	=	
Normal Values pocketcard		x	US $ 3.95	=	
Periodic Table pocketcard		x	US $ 3.95	=	
Psychiatry pocketcard		x	US $ 3.95	=	
Regional Anesthesia pocketcard Set (3)		x	US $ 9.95	=	
Vision pocketcard		x	US $ 3.95	=	

Books and Pocketcards also available at...   www.media4u.com